THE HISTORY AND POLITICS
OF COMMUNITY MENTAL HEALTH

THE
HISTORY AND POLITICS
OF
COMMUNITY MENTAL
HEALTH

MURRAY LEVINE

State University of New York at Buffalo

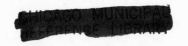
New York   Oxford
OXFORD UNIVERSITY PRESS
1981

Copyright © 1981 by Oxford University Press, Inc.

Library of Congress Cataloging in Publication Data

Levine, Murray, 1928-
    The history and politics of community mental health.

    Bibliography: p.
    Includes index.
    1. Community mental health services—United States—
History.   2. Mental health services—United States—His-
tory.   3. Mental health policy—United States—History.
4. Mental health services—Law and legislation—United
States.   I. Title. [DNLM: 1. Psychiatry, Community—
History—United States.   2. Community mental health
centers—History—United States.   3. Health policy—His-
tory—United States. WM 11 AA1 L6h]
RA790.6.L49   362.2′0973   81-1113
ISBN 0-19-502955-0   AACR2
ISBN 0-19-502956-9 (pbk.)

Printing (last digit): 987654321

Printed in the United States of America

To my wife Adeline,
who rightly said I became smart
after she studied sociology,
and to our two sons,
David and Zachary,
who have always been at the center
of our joint lives.

CONTENTS

THE HISTORY AND POLITICS
OF COMMUNITY MENTAL HEALTH

INTRODUCTION

Every mental health worker is aware of the concepts of community mental health, whether employed in the community mental health centers that were created to implement the concepts; employed in an improved inpatient institution (twenty years ago so widely condemned because of their inadequacies); or because theory and practice has been changed by the concepts underlying community based practice (e.g. crisis and support networks). While the viewpoint that I have elsewhere termed "intrapsychic supremacy" (the viewpoint that people's troubles stem from perceptions and reactions largely determined by internal psychological events; (Levine, 1969; 1970) is alive and well in the conceptual armamentarium of professional mental health workers, it has at least been leavened by the influence of sociological, situational and ecological viewpoints emphasizing the contributions of the social order to problems in living.

Today, one can engage in a good argument about the merits of labelling theory, for example, in describing the helpers' possible contribution to the pathology they seek to alleviate (see, for example, Scheff, 1966; Gove, 1970; Rosenhan, 1973, 1975; and his critics: Crown, 1975; Millon, 1975; Spitzer, 1975; Weiner, 1975), and everyone will understand the terms of the debate. Twenty years ago, few professional mental health workers would have known there was an issue, much less be prepared to engage in sophisticated argument. The coming of the community mental health movement, marked by President John F. Kennedy's mes-

sage to the Congress and by the Community Mental Health
Centers Act of 1963, left indelible impressions on the whole field,
even though one may argue about the true extent to which practice
has been affected.

The community mental health movement also marked the
entry of the federal government into the support of service delivery to an unprecedented extent. Before that time, the federal
government had provided some mental health support and services, particularly through Veterans Administration hospitals,
clinics, and training programs, and through the research and
training programs of the National Institute of Mental Health
(NIMH). In an earlier day, few were concerned about the federal
involvement because it was based on a philosophy of providing
resources to the field at large—to universities, medical schools,
research institutes, and to clinics and hospitals—for the necessary
training and research.

Federal policy from 1946 to 1961 can best be described as
supporting the growth of the mental health fields with little
attempt to exercise control over the direction of growth. To be
sure psychiatry was supported more handsomely than psychology,
social work, or nursing, and research with a biological core was
supported more generously than research grounded in psychological, sociological, or humanistic concepts and methods. The political nature of those judgments, in the sense that one area of work
was supported more handsomely and thus valued more than
another, was supported by the professional consensus on their
legitimacy. For about twenty-five years, from the beginnings of
NIMH in 1946 to the beginning of the 1970s, the mental health
fields were in an unprecedented period of growth, with little to
slow the increase in funds and number of professional people
working in the field.

Mental health politics in the 1950s was for the most part
limited to the issue of who was entitled to practice psychotherapy.
It would *not* have included the allocation and distribution of
funds for services. Most of the money came from state governments and was allocated through the byzantine processes of state
government. Some funds coming from the United Way were
allocated to their traditional agencies. Undoubtedly state commissioners of mental health were aware of the politics of dealing

with governors and legislatures, and undoubtedly agency executives were well aware of the fine points of the care and feeding of boards, and the politics of charities. But these concerns did not filter down to most line mental health workers, who felt little affected. There was very little professional self-consciousness about the politics of mental health.

The federal government was a cornucopia pouring forth unlimited resources and unlimited opportunities for growth and expansion. It did not appear to be exerting a force in any direction. Training grants were given to institutions to develop their own programs, subject only to general professional standards established by accrediting agencies. Research funds were given to scientists to support the research that scientists decided they wanted to do. These funds were dispersed by peer review groups based on a proposal's scientific merit, almost irrespective of its content. At least that's the way it appeared to professionals in the field.

The trend away from the state hospital as the major therapeutic resource and toward community based services was not clearly signalled by anything that came before. NIMH's success in meeting the growth needs of the field gave it a well deserved aura of competence and earned it respect in Congress and among professional leaders. The report of the congressionally commissioned Joint Commission on Mental Illness and Health set some new directions. With Kennedy-Johnson era support for the reform of social institutions, a more explicit and formal policy emerged to reduce the census of our mental institutions.

President Kennedy's Message to Congress on February 5, 1963, formally stated the aims of deinstitutionalizing and of providing community based care. (He also spoke of creating preventive programs, but the time for this idea had not yet come.) Few were aware at the time what a radical departure from previous policy this statement was. From that time on, it became clearer that the days of undirected growth were ending and the federal government was going to use its vast power to spend to promote its view of what the nation required in mental health. In time, funding for services was determined more and more by the requirements of the community mental health program. Policies governing the allocation of training funds and research funds also shifted, albeit slowly, to coincide with that major policy thrust, and to ensure that the training and research communities conformed to the aims of federal mental health policy. The professional lives of many were now to be directly affected by the flow of funds.

No social reform takes place in isolation. When one social institution is subject to the zeitgeist of change, it is probably true that others are as well (Levine & Levine, 1970). It does not follow, however, that because social reforms do not take place in isolation from each other, they take place in a planned and coordinated fashion. While there may be a general air of reform, it is characteristic of our government and of American society that there is a separation and dispersion of powers among the legislative, the executive, and the judiciary; among federal, state and local governments; between the public and private sectors; and between nodes of influence and power within each of those areas. While some have the power to order, or to influence others, the others, having independent power bases, also have the power to resist, or to use or to redirect resources to pursue their own priorities. It also does not follow that agencies of government, even at the same level, necessarily communicate with each other, much less cooperate.

Even though the problem of those served by our public mental health institutions may be characterized as a welfare problem and as a problem of social dependence, reforms in the funding of welfare and in the funding of health care went on parallel to reforms in the mental health service delivery system, but independent of them. Independently developed reforms did not come together until those responsible for administering institutions and services began using the fiscal tools available to pursue their own agencies' aims. Reforms then came together, but frequently not in ways that were predicted, or worse, in ways that were undesirable from the viewpoint of patient care. The short-lived Mental Health Systems Act (1980) was partly directed toward solving problems that were created by earlier legislative solutions to still earlier existing problems. If we have learned anything, it is that the slogan "Problem Creation Through Problem Solution" is very apt.

As recently as fifteen years ago, few professional mental health workers were aware of the role lawyers, litigation, and the judiciary would play in their lives. A few may have been dimly aware of issues in malpractice because the post–World War II period was marked by a flowering of medical malpractice suits and large settlements. Malpractice insurance for mental health professionals was cheap; it was rare that mental patients brought, much less won, malpractice suits. Those who worked in public facilities probably had some awareness of commitment procedures, and the legal in limbo status of committed patients. Only a few saw it as a problem, Szasz (1963) being foremost amongst those who did.

The reform era of the 1960s brought forth young lawyers uninterested in ordinary commercial practice and desiring a piece of the reform action. As poverty law flowered in the 1960s, so did mental health law. Lawyers, operating from a number of bases, not the least one funded by NIMH to promote institutional reform (Kopolow et al., 1975), and supported by a judiciary then open to enlightenment by psychiatrists and social scientists, attacked a number of misuses of mental health services in the criminal justice system, and a little bit later in civilian mental hospitals. Chapters 5 and 6 here are devoted to descriptions of the thrust and the impact of litigation (and some subsequent legislation) on mental hospital practices. Some of the most powerful and dramatic of reforms have been accomplished through litigation, but institutional resistance to change has defeated or modified the victories won in court. No matter the outcome, the line mental health worker's life has been influenced by the operation of our legal system, and one cannot fully understand the contemporary mental health scene without examining that impact.

This book deals much more with politics and legislation than it does with the substantive theories and findings of the community mental health movement. Chapter 7 centers on the report of the President's Commission on Mental Health (1978), tracing the impact of that report and its recommendations on the Mental Health Systems Act of 1980, a major piece of legislation intended to replace the Community Mental Health Centers Act. The chapter asserts that the predominant constituency for mental health services, training, and research funds, is now the providers of service. The providers are organized into professional groups, each pursuing its own aims. It is these aims, and the political issues behind them, that must be carefully examined, as the presence and activities of such organized groups will give shape to future mental health funding.

In the past our political, social, economic, and historical contexts—the ground against which our professional and scientific work was figure—went unnoticed. Our social world was organized reasonably to allow us to work as we chose. The fish, as the sage said, would be the last to discover water. We did not examine our contexts because they supported our professional lives. In recent years, however, the contexts have been invaded. What was our life support system, our "water," has been "polluted" by unworthy and irrational professional politics. The bureaucrats, lawyers, budget people, legislators, organizations, citizens who participate and protest, blacks, hispanics, asiatics, American Indians, ethnic Americans, women, and journalists exposing the deficiencies of deinstitutionalization and uncovering nursing home scandals have all become active parts of our professional contexts, influencing our day to day professional lives. Whether we have jobs or not, whether the services we render are reimbursible or not, whether or not we can get funding for our research or our training programs, whether we work within the walls of an institution or in a community based setting, are now determined by choate and inchoate governmental policies and less by professional wisdom about what sort of services we wish to provide, what kind of training we wish to do, and what sort of research problems we undertake.

One audience for this book is the line mental health worker who has suffered through the vagaries of policy and politics and the uncertainties of funding. What the line worker has experienced may have given him or her ulcers, or may have been experienced as irrational; however, the processes can be seen as systematic and inherent in our political and social system. This book is designed to give the professional mental health worker some distance from day to day problems and to provide some basis for understanding what happened, and how and why it happened.

This book is also directed to the student of community psychology and community mental health, social and community psychiatry, psychiatric nursing, social work, rehabilitation, public administration and policy, and mental health administration. When I was in graduate school, there was no such field as community psychology, and few professionals had any institutional ambitions beyond becoming a full professor or a director of psychological services. The thought that as professionals we had to concern ourselves with the social and political context of services, training, and research was foreign, and at the time would have seemed irrelevant. However, many students now in graduate training will influence future policy decisions and implement policy decisions in leadership roles and in their professional capacities. Once we acknowledge that our environment is a political one, it is necessary to understand the political game thoroughly. This book is not about politics in the sense that *Plunkitt of Tammany Hall* (Riordan, 1905) is about politics. However, I hope this book will help those students who enter leadership roles to understand what they have to understand to make sense of their professional roles. I also hope it will encourage the aspirations of some to accept leadership in the professional political context, and to see that participation can be in the public interest. Politics is not wrong or bad. It is inevitable. It is bad or wrong only if we blind ourselves to those inevitabilities.

Many of my ideas were stimulated by discussions with my wife Adeline, a sociologist, and with Seymour Sarason, and by his writings. Sarason (1981) has rightly berated American psychology for its unidimensional emphasis on the psychology of the individual. His complaint can be directed against other mental health fields with equal justice. This book is in support of his complaint. It is to say to students that we need to learn to think holistically if we are to deal with problems that we select but that are often enough thrust upon us.

Having said what this book is about, it is important to say what it is not about. It is *not* in any sense a definitive history based on research in primary sources. Almost everything is based on secondary sources, published research, and published government reports and statistics. I have not attempted to interview participants or to review documents to understand the story from the inside. This book is more an interpretation than it is a history of movements and people. The interpretations are grounded in sources I accept as reliable, but neither the reader (nor the writer) should confuse an imposed coherence with social reality. The social world is ordered, certainly, but it can be viewed from many different perspectives. I will defend my interpretation and my perspective, but I recognize that others may see the issues quite differently. The word *history* in the title may claim too much.

The book does not deal with the growth and differentiation of the National Institute of Mental Health as a political organization. Someone seeking a discussion of the development of institutes for drug abuse or alcohol, or of the various organizational locations of NIMH itself within Health, Education and Welfare, or of the considerations leading to the development of the Alcohol, Mental Health and Drug Abuse Administration (ADAMHA) will seek in vain. I have not covered those issues because they did not seem directly related to the themes I was trying to develop. They are important, and my story may be less precise because of the omission.

I have not discussed prominent actors in the mental health drama. My aim was to sketch in the interaction of programs and events, and to highlight those interactions. It is not that I believe that history is better told as a history of events, rather than a history of actors. I have not given up on psychology. I am convinced there is a person-environment interaction, and that some persons are better prepared and better able to take advantage of events than others. My story is poorer and less precise because of those omissions. I do not say that to excuse this work's shortcomings, but rather to tell my readers what I intended, and what they will and will not find in the book.

Finally, the reader cannot help but note that my presentation is by no means neutral. I have tried to signal my personal views and my personal feelings as best I could. The book may contain more moralizing than many readers will find warranted, or even seemly. The issues are, though, in many ways moral issues, and require the exercise of a moral sentiment. I have participated only in small ways in some of the programs that I wrote about. I am not an expert in history, political science, legislation, litigation, or the practice of community mental health. I am a professor of psychology, based in a university. The book's merits and deficiencies reflect the freedom provided by my home base to think and write about what I thought was important. I have written as I have because others have not and because I found this a useful way to think. I hope my readers will also find the perspective useful.

Chapter 1

CARE OF THE MENTALLY ILL
Change in Historical Context

The state and county mental hospital, the primary element of the system of care for so many years before the onset of community mental health programs, had its own precursors. As an institution, it was designed to meet the problems of its day and was shaped for the future by forces not anticipated by its designers. In this chapter, I shall examine the origins of that care system, explore the ways in which it evolved, the ways in which it failed the purposes of its designers, and the forces involved. This exploration of history is useful in its own right, to provide some perspective on an intractable problem. However, it is also useful because historical perspective helps us to identify some of the elements of the elaborate social and political context that shaped the hospital in its time. By teasing out those elements we may be able to alert ourselves to analogous forces that influence modern efforts to provide care to similarly situated groups of people.

Early care in Europe. In one way or another, civilization has always recognized its madmen and made provision to deal with them. The variety of themes of madness are well developed by Rosen (1968), who makes the point that in the discussions of what constitutes illness and how to care for those afflicted, one can see the premises of the society which defines, interprets, and classifies behavior and people as deviant. Depressives and violent individuals who acted in impulsive, uncontrolled, and unreasonable ways were always recognized as mad. While various cultures looked upon the causes of these behaviors differently, some thread of possession by evil spirits, demonic influences, or the baleful influence of the gods was a common explanation through the middle ages. In the seventeenth and eighteenth centuries with the rise of a mercantile society, a capitalistic class, and scientific reasoning, a concept of losing rationality became more prominent. The definition of mental illness came to include crimes against property as well as propriety. A son heavily in debt and discharged from the army in disgrace, or the mistress of a bourgeois gentleman who had enticed him to spend his fortune on her, could be committed as mad. Drunkenness, profanity, blasphemy and even overreligiosity came to be considered offenses against the stable social order and could lead to incarceration.

Generally, madmen who were not too troublesome were tolerated and allowed to wander about. If they were too troublesome, they were driven away from their communities. Sometimes they were turned over to boatmen who left them in some distant place. In some places there were religious institutions, or places of care in monasteries or convents. Mad people were organized into pilgrimages to religious shrines. Foucault (1965) points out that the Ship of Fools, a theme in the painting and literature of the middle ages, represented cargoes of madmen in search of their reason and perhaps reflected some organized effort on their behalf. Madness, Foucault says, was not a prominent problem until the last part of the fifteenth century. Before that time death and disease were the focus of literature and art.

Toward the end of the Middle Ages, from the thirteenth century onward, scholars claim that a sense of melancholy and pessimism marked the times, attributed to perceptions that the world was changing. Many in that time felt that madness was on the increase, a sign of the end of the world. As western civilization moved out of feudalism, with its tightly ordered world, into the mercantile era, where authority relations were changing, madness became a theme of growing interest. Rosen (1968) points to the sixteenth and seventeenth century characters of Don Quixote, King Lear, and Ophelia as representative of that era's concern with madness.

Until the end of the Middle Ages, communities were able to tolerate a few madmen wandering around, and it could even support them to some extent. However, as a consequence of social and political change, the breakdown of feudal estates, and religious wars, with struggles for authority among the contending groups, a large disaffected class was created in France and in England. Foucault estimates that in a population of 100,000 in mid-seventeenth century Paris, there were 30,000 paupers—the unemployed, disbanded soldiers, impoverished students, the sick, and the insane. The French Parliament in 1656 authorized a huge place of confinement, the Hopital Generale, in which beggars, indigents, vagrants, the unemployed, the sick, and the insane were confined and put to work, in part as a means of controlling a social crisis.

Similar processes were ongoing in England. Peasants had been driven off the lands, forcing huge migrations of rural people into the cities in search of employment. In consequence a large and permanent pauper class was created. Attempts to deal with the problems of poverty went on sporadically until the development of the Elizabethan poor laws in 1601. These formalized the concept of local community responsibility for the poor. Each parish provided an overseer of the poor, who had to provide for care. The law made individuals responsible for their kin and it allowed commitment to a house of correction for those who would not work. If nothing more, these laws established a tradition that the community had a corporate responsibility for the poor and the dependent (Deutsch, 1949).

In England, with the developing industrial revolution and a rapidly rising population (England and Wales increased in population from 7 million to 12 million between 1760 and 1820, during the reign of George III), there was further movement off the land. Moreover the substitution of machinery for hand labor led to a drastic reorganization of life styles. From 1815 to 1830 there were frequent working-class riots, the consequence of problems people were experiencing at that time. Historians are in general agreement that the industrial revolution consolidated the large pauper class, and it was here that the great rise in lunacy was noted (Parry-Jones, 1972).

Throughout the eighteenth century, lunatic hospitals were opened in cities all over England, supplementing the system of boarding madmen in licensed private madhouses or in private homes. The York Retreat was opened in 1796 by the Society of Friends in reaction to the poor care available in existing institutions. It was there that William Tuke did his work in establishing the moral therapy which was to become so influential in the United States (Parry-Jones, 1972).

The eighteenth century was also the age of enlightenment, when science had all but replaced religious authority in defining knowledge and truth. The late eighteenth century also saw the French Revolution, bringing social upheaval. The age of science, coming as it did in tandem with a profound revolution in social thought, provided the context in which Phillippe Pinel opened the gates of the Bicêtre and the Salpêtrière, two major hospitals in Paris, and removed the chains from the mad men and women who had been kept in dungeons because they were unable to work and were threatening to their keepers and others. Perhaps foreshadowing modern experience, Pinel demonstrated that the predictions of violence were unwarranted. With a combination of kindness and firmness he was able to treat many thought hopeless and to help them to improve. His writings (Pinel, 1806) were translated and were influential in the United States.[1]

One other factor is worthy of note. King George III, apparently given to depressive episodes, was hospitalized four times during his long reign. The King's hospitalizations called attention to mental illness, and in the course of a Parliamentary inquiry into his treatment (the royal personage had been abused by an attendant, with the consent of his physician), the physician, who maintained a private asylum, claimed that he cured nine out of every ten mental patients he treated. A few years later other proprietors of private institutions, not to be outdone, made similar claims, helping to create what has been called the cult of curability (Deutsch, 1949). Apparently, mental illness took on a certain fashionableness for patients and physicians, given that it was a royal illness (Caplan, 1969). Szasz (1961) has noted that it was necessary to recast mental problems into a medical model in order to justify humane treatment of the mentally disordered.

1. Jean-Baptiste Pussin, an unlettered paraprofessional who was governor of the insane at the Bicêtre, was Pinel's tutor and indeed many of Pinel's ideas and practices came from Pussin's work and from his unpublished manuscripts (Weiner, 1979).

Apparently, it was also necessary to claim miracles to obtain public attention and to claim public resources.

The United States. Very similar processes could be observed in the United States. During the colonial period, through the eighteenth century, neither pauperism nor insanity was a critical problem. The colonies accepted the English principle that it was the responsibility of local communities to care for their own. Since colonial society was predominantly rural, deviant behavior was largely tolerated. In sparsely settled areas, persons who broke social rules could easily keep to themselves. People could work in relative isolation and labor was scarce. Dangerous individuals would be incarcerated, sometimes in jails, and sometimes in individual cages or pens on family property, but paid for by the community. Wealthier families kept their deranged members in attics or cellars and hired private attendants. Paupers were often sold at auction to the lowest bidder, who agreed to care for them at the lowest price. The bidder was allowed to work those in his charge. The insane and the feebleminded who were not too uncontrollable were thus in some demand. Demented individuals who were not dangerous wandered about and generally were "warned out" of town so they should not become a local responsibility. Apparently it was not unknown for one community's officials to spirit away a demented person in the middle of the night and dump that individual on another town's doorstep. However, with population growth, these informal community-based means for caring for the insane and the indigent failed and institutions were built. Boston established an almshouse in 1662 in which the poor, the aged, the blind, the insane, idiots, and orphans were confined together. Other cities followed suit. Some built workhouses in which the individual's greeting was ten lashes (Deutsch, 1949).

The scientific spirit however, was prominent in the United States as well as in Europe. The Pennsylvania Hospital opened a ward for lunatics in 1752, albeit in the basement, and although there were attempts to treat patients medically, especially under the influence of Benjamin Rush, some of the treatment of the day, purging, blistering the skin, bleeding, and other shock tactics, appear rather punitive from a modern perspective. Virginia opened the first institution devoted exclusively to the mentally ill in 1773 (Deutsch, 1949; Rothman, 1971; Grob, 1973).

By 1800 concentrations of population in the growing cities made the public much more aware of "queer" or deviant behavior. King George's fashionable malady and associated writings were known among Americans who traveled back and forth across the Atlantic. Boston had a population of 25,000 and was beginning to face the problems of an urban area. Moreover, by the early 1800s wealthy businessmen and merchants had begun giving large sums of money for charities in an effort to exemplify the concept that wealth was not for private benefit but for public good. In several places hospitals were built with such private subscriptions, often after a public drive supported by the clergy and the local press. A number of these hospitals, influenced by the possibilities for treatment which were spoken of in Europe, added psychiatric wards. In a democratic spirit, these hospitals were to accept all, but they were small institutions and their managers found ways of excluding the poor (Grob, 1966).

Moral therapy and its decline. The Worcester State Hospital in Massachusetts was built in growing awareness of the problems of the mentally ill, in a spirit of reform that led to the creation of a variety of institutions (Rothman, 1971) during the early part of the nineteenth century. The Worcester hospital was important because it was the first that was systematically designed for mental patients and it was the first to be supported by state funds exclusively. It was built as a therapeutic institution and served as a model, if not a training institution, for those who established hospitals elsewhere (e.g., see Gish, 1972). Built to implement the principles of moral therapy, the Worcester hospital declined in relatively few years. Its ideals were replaced by the dictum that insanity was incurable, a view that shaped mental hospital practices and policies from the middle of the nineteenth century onward.

Various commissions concerned with prison reform had called attention to the insane who were badly abused in jails, which were sometimes as primitive as an abandoned mine. In 1830 Horace Mann, the educator, a person typical of the intellectual reformer of the post-Jacksonian era, concerned with prison reform, abolition, and women's rights among other causes, chaired a Massachusetts legislative committee which completed a census of the insane. The commission believed there were 500 insane people in Massachusetts and recommended the establishment of a hospital for the insane. Citing European authorities Pinel and Tuke and experience at the earlier established Hartford Retreat in Connecticut under Eli Todd (Reisman, 1976), Mann argued that the insane could be cured, removing them from the welfare rolls and saving the state money in the long run. If the breadwinner of a family was ill, the whole family fell into poverty, so treatment had important potential not only for rehabilitating the sick person but also for saving the community the cost of caring for that person's family as well. American optimism denied there was a permanent pauper class here, so a therapeutic solution to the problems of individuals seemed warranted (Grob, 1966).

Some believe the arguments may have been overstated deliberately in order to sell the legislature on a hospital, or it may simply have been enthusiasm and lack of data that led to the extravagant claims. At any rate, when the claims that hospitals cured and saved money were not borne out, a serious backlash caused therapeutic ideals to be subordinated to cost-conscious custodial care (Grob, 1966; 1973). That story will be told below.

For now, let us note that a problem came to public attention as a result of social change which made former means of caring for the afflicted and the dependent inadequate. An intellectual climate of reform, and optimism, based more on ideology than close examination of hard facts led to the adoption of a solution by government. The solution became embedded in the complexities of the political and the social order and that context was to shape the fate of efforts to care for the mentally ill for the next 100 years.

A hospital was opened in 1833 in Worcester, a town of 4200, about 40 miles from Boston. Centrally located, rail and stage lines passed through it. The then governor of Massachusetts was a Worcester resident and the town legislature voted $2500 to purchase a site (Grob, 1966). It is obvious that the area benefited from construction contracts and employment,[2] although available

---

2. To this day, there are many communities that are largely dependent upon their prisons, mental hospitals and other institutions for employment and for local business. Moves to take patients out of the institutions and to close them sometimes meet with strong political opposition for such reasons (Levine, 1980).

histories say little about this. In later years, reformers in other states would point with horror to the "pauper's palaces" and "lunatic cathedrals" that were built with public monies by politically favored contractors (Deutsch, 1949). Once the hospital became a public facility, its character was shaped by the political process.

Moral therapy and many other institutional reforms took hold in the post-Jacksonian era. Andrew Jackson was the first non-aristocrat to attain the Presidency. His election in 1829 was symbolic of a changing social order. A new elite arose, its wealth coming from trade and factories rather than from land and agriculture. Observers of that day believed that an older, more graceful life was giving way to the unbridled pursuit of wealth and material advantage (Tucker, 1855). There were profound shifts in well settled legal doctrine in civil law in favor of economic development, undermining expectations about property rights, and undermining the paternal relationship between employer and employee (Horwitz, 1977). Religious reform, educational change, prison reform, women's rights, abolitionist efforts, and temperance movements all arose during these times. A variety of utopianisms spread over the land during the next fifty years (Levine & Bunker, 1975). Charles Finney's revivalist crusade held Rochester, New York, in its fervent grip for six months beginning in September of 1830, then it spread west to towns in Ohio and Michigan and east to Utica, Albany, and to towns in New England, even affecting sophisticated New York City and Philadelphia. Johnson (1978) argues the revivals took hold as a means of imposing social control, and as a means of restoring cohesiveness to communities badly rent by social and economic change. Looking back wistfully on the simple agrarian society as the ideal, commentators believed there was an actual increase in mental disorder as a result of social and economic dislocations caused by technological, economic, and social change (Caplan, 1969).

Given the theory that insanity and other social problems were caused by the changing social order, it made sense to try to treat the insane by modifying the social order of the institutional environment. In theory, the deranged person could be restored to sanity by living in a sane environment, the asylum. That the institution served to stabilize the social order by removing deviants may not have been fully apparent to thinkers of that day. American concepts of individualism supported beliefs in the responsibility of individuals for their own plights. Treatment was directed toward changing the individual rather than toward removing the ultimate cause by changing the larger social environment (Rothman, 1971).

Samuel Woodward, the first superintendent of Worcester, had had experience in moral therapy at the Hartford Retreat in Connecticut, under Eli Todd. A distinguished physician, Woodward had been active in several reform movements of the day. A religious man, he shared with many reformers an abiding faith in the perfectibility of people, in the concept of perpetual human progress, and eventually in human ability to create a utopia on earth. Apparently an irrepressible optimist, he had great faith that evil could be overcome with good and that no matter an individual's condition, he or she could be helped.

In keeping with the associationist psychology of the time developed by Locke, Hume, and Hartley, Woodward believed that insanity was a disease of the brain but that the mind, somewhat like the soul, was incorporeal and could never become permanently diseased. Believing that knowledge came to the mind only through the senses, he argued that if the therapist could control and manipulate the environment, providing the patient with new and different stimuli, older undesirable patterns of association could be broken and newer ones substituted in their place. Some may see forerunners of the therapeutic environment and of the Skinnerian concept of stimulus control in Woodward's theory (Grob, 1966).

The theory was implemented by a regime of regular living, a simple but substantial diet, an emphasis on personal cleanliness, occupational therapy, religious exercises, reading, amusements, and sports. In a typical day, Woodward and his assistant physician saw every patient in his or her room, spoke to each one, inquired of the patient's needs, and suggested work or recreation. Woodward's assistant physician was on the wards directly in contact with patients. Attendants, trained by the superintendent, reported directly to him. Woodward said that the essence of the treatment program resided in the close relationship established between staff and patients. Kindness was coupled with firmness, but the expectations the staff held out for the patients were critical:

> If there is any secret in the management of the insane, it is this: respect them and they will respect themselves; treat them as reasonable beings and they will take every possible pains to show you that they are such; give them your confidence, and they will rightly appreciate it and rarely abuse it. (in Grob, 1966, p. 66.)

Woodward's results were from all reports excellent and comparable to the best results of modern day institutions. While in later times other authors questioned the validity of statistics reported by mental hospitals, Woodward was discharging fifty percent or more of his patients and they stayed out of the hospital in goodly numbers. Later on, at the Worcester hospital and in other hospitals, results became progressively poorer, until in the latter part of the nineteenth century, the American psychiatrist Pliny Earle pronounced the insane incurable. Discharge rates dropped further after that (Bockoven, 1972).

Grob (1973) presents data on hospitals that filed annual reports from the earliest days through 1875. Taking the number discharged as recovered as a percentage of the number of admissions that year, I obtained a median discharge rate of 46 percent for hospitals in 1840. That had dropped to a median of 30 percent by 1875. Eleven of 15 institutions for which Grob reported data showed the decline. What happened to change the results and professional attitudes toward mental illness after propitious beginnings?

Chronic patients. First, moral therapists overestimated the power of the treatment methods they employed. The best results were claimed for recent cases. But when even a small percentage failed to recover, hospital facilities eventually became swamped with the failures of treatment. Hospital superintendents made valiant efforts to conceal these difficulties and manipulated their statistics. Cures were claimed as a percentage of those discharged and not as a percentage of those admitted. Those that died were included among the successes. Cases were reclassified as new or old, depending on whether they improved, and were counted accordingly. The chronic patient became a threat to be concealed and was not looked at as a problem to be confronted in its own right. Hospital superintendents manipulated their statistics either to press their claims for more resources, or simply to keep up their professional reputations (Caplan, 1969).

Second, the hospitals were inundated, not with the treatable, early cases, but with the most troublesome and dangerous individuals who were incarcerated in local facilities. A third of the first 164 patients had been confined under poor conditions for periods varying from 10 to 32 years. Eight of the first 40 inmates were murderers. The figures used by Horace Mann to assess need soon proved inadequate. Although there was some knowledge of the number of patients in jails and the like, the need assessment did not anticipate that families, seeing the hospital as a resource that would help their family members, sent their relatives there rather than keep them home. Demand quickly outstripped capacity. From 1830 to 1850 the population of Massachusetts rose 63 percent, while the population of the Worcester hospital rose from 107 in 1833 to 359 in 1846, without, of course, a concomitant increase in resources (Grob, 1966).

Laws governing admission. While involuntary commitment was accomplished through a rather simple and informal process, the law establishing the hospital required that it admit the "furiously mad" and the criminally insane. Hospital officials had no control over these admissions. The law also required that local communities pay for any of their pauper residents who were sent to the hospital. Local communities were reluctant to send any but their most troublesome citizens since it was considerably cheaper to maintain people in the almshouses and workhouses than to pay the fees charged by the state hospital. The provisions of the law guaranteed that the hospital would develop an image as a place where hopeless public menaces were incarcerated.

Given that reputation, middle-class clients became ever more reluctant to send their relatives to the state institution. The wealthy used the prestigious private hospitals which excluded the poor, while the middle-class sought out less expensive proprietary institutions if they could afford them. A self-reinforcing process developed in which the state hospital eventually was viewed as a place for the poor and the dangerous (Grob, 1966; 1973). The laws did not include provision for increments in resources with increments in patient populations and as it became apparent that the hospitals were serving the poor, political willingness to commit resources declined.

Class, ethnic, and racial factors. While there had always been some discriminatory treatment between paying and nonpaying patients at the hospitals, the distinctions were rationalized on the grounds that a proper therapeutic environment should not require people who were obnoxious to each other to mingle. Blacks were either denied admission to hospitals or were housed in segregated facilities that were invariably poorer than those for pauper whites. People with different cultural backgrounds could not mingle easily and therapeutic considerations supported differential allocation of resources by class. Nevertheless, at first most patients were native Americans, part of the White Anglo-Saxon Protestant culture. Patients, although behaving in difficult, puzzling, frightening ways, were not seen as some lesser form of humanity (Grob, 1966; 1973).

Between 1847 and 1854, two and one half million immigrants entered the United States. About 40 percent of these were Irish Catholics. These foreigners, of different religious background, speaking a different language, and with differing cultural characteristics soon produced disproportionate numbers of mental patients, particularly in urban hospitals. The immigrants, who were dispossessed from their own lands by economic problems, were destitute. Irish Catholics provided the cheap labor for developing factories but they soon were seen to produce dirty, dangerous slums. Native Americans believed that their way of life was being ruined by a poor class of immigrants who were being shipped here by Europeans. Americans resented them for their Catholicism, for their different ways, for their different language, and for their dependence on the welfare roles. Very quickly, it was the immigrant who began to make up the hospital population, as many as 75 percent of all recent admissions in some institutions (Grob, 1966; 1973).

The Irish were seen as dirty, ignorant, jealous, drunken debauchers, victims of their own bad habits, not victims of social conditions, and unable to assimilate or to adjust to the American way of life. The native American staff felt they were not trusted by the Irish. The hospital superintendents who were all New Englanders or Northeasterners, Protestants, and college educated males couldn't communicate with the Irish. The cultural communalities between therapist and patient that underlay moral treatment apparently did not exist in the relationship between hospital personnel and their new clientele. A treatment based upon mutual expectations simply did not work. Moreover, given public attitudes toward the Irish, the influx of patients was not matched by an influx of resources. The influx of immigrant Irish in cultural conflict with native Americans contributed to the demise of moral therapy. Legislators became still less interested in expending resources on worthless foreigners who couldn't be helped in any event (Grob, 1966; 1973).

Professionalism, patronage, and hospital staff. Hospital superintendents were a rather homogenous group. Well-educated native Americans, the earlier individuals tended to be humanitarian reformers and men of wide interests and great abilities. Pay was relatively poor, but apparently the early superintendents accepted the positions out of interest and out of moral commitment. The second generation of hospital superintendents tended to be managers rather than reformers and were without the intellectual drive of their mentors. They saw it as their task to work with what they had. As hospitals filled with chronic patients and as legislators became more stinting in their appropriations, hospital superintendents turned to the development of the most efficient means of managing the masses of difficult patients in their institutions. Still hospital superintendents were interested in maintaining a professional self-image, and so they developed professional associations, which tended to be a closed corporation. The forerunner of the American Psychiatric Association was organized in 1844 and it cooperated in the publication of the American Journal of Insanity, the forerunner of the American Journal of Psychiatry. The professional organization served the several purposes such organizations do, but it also tended to be restrictive, closely controlling practices and standards. The hospital psychiatrists used their combined expertise as leverage to maintain their positions vis à vis the public and the legislators. Much of their battle was to maintain the autonomy of the superintendent as a medical expert.

With the emphasis on professional expertise, attendants were no longer viewed as part of the therapeutic team, but more as keepers of chronic clients. They received neither training nor interesting responsibilities. The positions were never well paid, and as employment in the institutions became less satisfying, staff shortages were frequent. Low-paying, unexciting, poor prestige jobs attracted a rather poor class of attendant, exacerbating the difficulties in maintaining a treatment orientation. In New York City criminals were assigned duties as mental hospital attendants (Grob, 1966; 1973). Moreover, hospital positions were treated as political patronage, with the result that local political figures attempted to influence the selection of superintendents, and especially the selection of aids. Personnel who owed their positions to political patrons were less responsive to hospital authority, with the result that care suffered still more (Gish, 1972).

The influence of reformers. The mid-nineteenth century continued to be a time marked by the activities of diverse reformers. None was more important to the system of care for the mentally ill than Dorothea Dix. A frail New England schoolmistress, she became interested in the problem of mental hospitals when teaching a Sunday school class in a jail. Identifying with those seeking to emancipate women from their sheltered roles, Dorothea Dix began a lifelong career to remove the insane from jails, alms-houses, and workhouses, where they were kept in abominable conditions, to the new mental hospitals. Her method was one of visiting every institution in a state, compiling vivid, detailed descriptions of the treatment of the insane and then "memorializing" state legislators in fiery speeches. Dedicated, determined, if not fanatical, Miss Dix buttonholed, bullied, and cajoled legislators until they would build additional hospital facilities. Over the course of her lifetime she was responsible for founding or enlarging 32 mental hospitals. While she was concerned with the proper care of the insane, Miss Dix was no theoretician, nor did she consider alternatives in care. She pressed forth singlemindedly to establish more hospitals (Deutsch, 1949).

Unusually successful in her activities, she became extremely influential, serving as a consultant to state legislatures who wished to improve their hospitals and as a recommender of superintendents of institutions. However, her vigorous activities led to still more admissions of difficult, chronic patients, adding to the reputations of hospitals as places for the poor and the dangerous. Moreover, since her concern was for the abuse of patients, critics felt her activities might have led to increased concern within hospitals with security, with more emphasis on rigid rules and on managerial efficiency, rather than upon active therapies (Bockoven, 1972). Be that as it may, it is undoubtedly true that the developing mental hospital movement owed much to Miss Dix's heroic efforts.

Another breed of critic emerged in mid-nineteenth century. Commitment laws were lax as we have noted. Not much more than a physician's signature was required to commit an individual in most places. It apparently became popular for some patients, upon release, to write books exposing abusive care, and charging that they and many others had been railroaded into mental hospitals. These works were popular and in some instances instigated legislative investigations of the hospitals. Mrs. Elizabeth Packard's book ([1875] 1973) was among the more influential of these works, and her efforts eventually led to some states requiring jury trials before an individual could be committed. (That development is discussed in Chapter 5 on litigation.) More importantly, the public accusations led hospital superintendents to feel they were under unfair attack. Many acted to exclude the public and to isolate their institutions still further from the community (Dain, 1964; Caplan, 1969; Grob, 1973).

Finally, in the third quarter of the nineteenth century, fiscal and managerial reformers appeared on the scene. Increasing welfare problems, the almshouses, those receiving other forms of relief and the rising costs of mental hospitals led reformers to press for centralized control of all welfare, including the hospitals. At first investigatory commissions were appointed, but soon these turned into powerful centralized agencies which wrested control of policy from local institutions. The issues were complex. They included the desire of public officials to end the wrangling between local and state authorities about who pays. They were based on a belief that local solutions failed, and that it would be possible to introduce cost-cutting managerial efficiency by centralizing control. Because funding for mental illness was grouped with attempts to find solutions for welfare problems, all of the negative attitudes associated with welfare were associated with mental hospitals and influenced the willingness to allocate resources to these institutions. Centralization left bureaucratization with all of its attendant complexities in managing human service institutions. Moreover, because the reformers were managerially oriented and were part of the scientific charity movement, budgetary standards of evaluation replaced therapeutic standards. Cost per capita became a more important criterion for evaluating hospitals than the quality of life within institutions, or even whether or not patients were helped by the institutions (Deutsch, 1949; Rothman, 1971; Grob, 1973).

Ideology and budgets. Mr. Dooley, a fictitious social and political commentator, once said he didn't know whether the flag followed the constitution, or the constitution followed the flag, but he surely believed the Supreme Court followed the election returns. Similarly, it is difficult to say whether ideology causes or follows given effects, but it is surely true that ideology arises in justification of what is. In the early years of the moral treatment movement, hospital superintendents published glowing reports of their successes, concealing failures and in effect denying that chronic patients were filling their institutions. As late as 1863, the annual report of the Worcester State Hospital emphasized the dollar value of benefits of treatment in the hospital of patients returned to a full life in the community (Caplan, 1969).

Pliny Earle is a well known name in mid-nineteenth century American psychiatry. An early advocate of moral treatment, he installed his version of it when he became superintendent of the Northampton Hospital in Massachusetts in 1864. Earle apparently ran a model institution, with a full therapeutic program. During his 21-year tenure as Superintendent, he never exceeded his budget, accumulating a cash surplus of $34,000. During his tenure the values of the state hospital grounds increased over 60 percent. The profit came from patient labor on the farm, and from careful management. Because he was able to reduce costs and show a profit, Earle was greatly admired by the profit-oriented businessmen who are so influential in our public affairs (Bockoven, 1972).

In contrast to an earlier generation of moral therapists who claimed high rates of cure, Earle eventually developed the concept that insanity was incurable. Discharge rates had been going down steadily for reasons we have described above. Superintendents had tended to adapt docilely to these conditions rather than fight them. The superintendents had made strong efforts to conceal the facts, but Earle carefully studied available statistics, pointed out their fallacies, and propounded the doctrine that insanity was incurable. His pronouncement was greeted with considerable relief by his contemporaries because he made it possible for them to accept the obvious fact that the cure rate was substantially under the 90 percent that had been promised initially.

Bockoven (1972) has carefully reanalyzed the available data, and it is his conclusion that the discharge rate was not nearly as bad as Earle insisted. Bockoven believed that a rate of about 50 percent was justified for the moral therapies, but the lower overall rate, in the face of greater promise, was looked upon as extreme failure, and led to the view that insanity was incurable.

Bockoven believes that there is evidence showing a connection between a high proportion of working patients, low discharge rates, and the excellent financial condition of Earle's hospital. Earle's biographer said:

> It was to this steady but not compulsory discipline of labor that the financial success of the hospital was due in great part; and though the record at Northampton showed small numbers . . . there were many unrecorded *virtual* recoveries—patients who, while still insane, were capable of self-support and self-direction under kindly supervision. (F.B. Sanborn, quoted in Bockoven, 1972, pp. 52–53)

In other words, the financial status of the hospital and the cost of care superceded the cure rate as an index of effectiveness. Cure rates were subordinated to discharge rates, and less effort was made to discharge patients. Bockoven states that discharge rates declined to under 20 percent in the 1920s and frequently fell as low as 5 percent. While not all hospitals turned a profit, the ideological justification for retaining patients meshed neatly with the value of having experienced laborers operating state hospital facilities. To what extent such a profit motive kept patients from being discharged cannot be estimated. However, it is worth noting that the theory of insanity propounded by Earle, and accepted by his contemporaries, fit very well with the emphasis on reducing costs of hospital care.

Grob (1973) also points out that the superintendents of that time rarely experimented with alternative modes of care, although plans for such were discussed from time to time. The leading hospital superintendents tended to reject such plans as ineffective and as more costly than what was in existence. The hospital superintendents generally desired smaller institutions at scattered locations throughout each state, although over the years, the number of patients considered desirable for a small institution crept up. It is not clear that hospital superintendents were so motivated, but that particular solution, at a minimum, would have created more hospitals, and coincidentally more hospital superintendencies. Alternatives that did not enhance the power of the profession were routinely rejected.

The large institution, housing growing numbers of chronic patients, a conglomeration of social rejects, and discharging few on the theory that insanity was incurable, persisted as the primary element in the system of mental health care until well after the Second World War. The last vestiges of moral therapy disappeared from the state and local hospitals, not to reappear until after World War II.

Some observations. This historical survey should remind us that we have long had a dependent population that has produced a disproportionate share of people classed as social problems. The informal means of care worked to some extent, but unregulated care was frequently brutal . . . and in the end unsuccessful. Placing responsibility for care of the dependent population in local hands proved unsatisfactory because local governments did not have the necessary resources, and in any event were reluctant to use their resources for the care of the dependent. Today we see that local governments, particularly in those states which have more generous welfare benefits, are encountering more and more voter resistance to using local taxes for welfare purposes. The Community Mental Health Act (see Chapter 2) envisioned placing increasing responsibility for the mentally ill and the mentally retarded in the hands of local communities, on the assumption that local responsibility would lead to more loving care. Historical precedent would suggest that in the absence of adequate resources, no such objective will be achieved. We may be going around in historical circles, simply because we do not pay serious attention to history.

We also noted that welfare problems and mental health problems are inextricably intertwined. When we examine care in the modern day, we will find much the same continues to hold true. County poor farms, almshouses, and workhouses persisted into the 1930s, and continued to have a mixture of clientele. It is ironic that when social security legislation was passed in 1935, the Act specifically excluded those in institutions from receiving its benefits. Those who thought of the problems said the infirm could be handled in state hospitals (Levine, 1979). In the post–World War II days, as we shall see in the next chapter, it was the aged who were the first targets of efforts to empty state hospitals, because they didn't belong there. We shall also see that fragmenting responsibility for welfare agencies for the mentally ill, for the retarded, for the aged, for the handicapped, and for the dependent, and into agencies for income maintenance, agencies for treatment, and agencies for housing created as many problems as it solved. The most cursory examination of historical trends brings that problem home to us.

Once considerations of care entered the political domain, a variety of vested interests made their weight felt in the actions that eventually emerged. In this case, local communities, the class interests of different segments of society, political usages of monies and jobs, and efforts of professional groups to enlarge or to protect turfs can all be identified. We can also identify intriguing issues by comparing the social characteristics of those who fulfill helping roles and the characteristics of those they help. If the difference in language and culture is at all marked, then actors who should relate closely and sympathetically may be alienated from each other. Moral therapy, which depended upon mutual trust and the fulfillment of mutual expectations, failed when cultural preconditions for mutuality were not met. The historical precedent requires us to raise questions about the cultural characteristics of helpers and those they help as critical variables affecting service delivery (see Levine & Levine, 1970).

The historical example warns us that fashions and fads in treatment, based on inadequate data, somehow attain cultural status as validated wisdom, and these ideas influence public policy. Proponents of new fashions in treatment tend to oversell them, to overpromise results, and to minimize difficulties. Public officials seeking solutions to intractable problems are often influenced more by enthusiasms than by carefully evaluated information, and will generalize the solution to problems it was never meant to solve; and by committing insufficient resources they will guarantee failure. Sometimes hard-pressed public officials will adopt professional rhetoric for their own purposes, and professionals, for their own reasons, cooperate in producing ideologies in justification of what is. Public policy is established with inadequate data, inadequate understanding of key issues, and with unrealistic expectations. Excess baggage may be added to a program for expedient reasons, and when failures are revealed, ad hoc solutions develop with long-range consequences that are unclear at the time, but which fix a course alterable only with grave difficulty.

The social sciences, inappropriately following the physical sciences, tend to be ahistorical. Social scientists assume, incorrectly, that contemporary developments are constructive and progressive outgrowths of previously tested knowledge. Social science does not procede linearly from a base of previously established knowledge, and on the basis of well validated, current findings. Applications of social science are intimately tied to the social order and shaped much more by the social and political contexts of the time than by powerful technologies derived from well tested theory (Levine & Levine, 1970). Our brief glimpse of history should, at the very least, alert us to the political and social context in which developments in social science thinking are nurtured. Our methods of care for those of our fellow citizens we come to call our patients reflect much more than just the experience, the thinking, and the study of those charged with their care. Our methods of care and our thinking are intimately interwoven into the fabric of society. If we look at just the warp or the woof, we will miss the design.

Chapter 2

MENTAL HEALTH
AND THE FEDERAL GOVERNMENT
The Earliest Steps

From 1830 to 1945, there were no real developments in mental health services affecting the general public. To be sure, services for children developed around the turn of the century (Levine & Levine, 1970), but aside from the creation of the psychopathic hospital (basically a mental hospital for short-term care, located in urban communities), there was not much else. The state hospital, which had been established with such high hopes, had fairly well run its course by the 1870s, and aside from some development in treatment technology in the 1930s (e.g., electroshock treatment, insulin shock, and later, lobotomies [Reisman, 1976]), the state hospital continued to be the mainstay of the mental health service system.

The provision of care for most mental health problems is the responsibility of state and local government, given the traditions and the divisions of responsibility in our federal system. However, in recent years, particularly after World War II, the major initiatives in mental health, and especially for community based services have come from the federal government. From one viewpoint, federal involvement in mental health is quite remarkable because the federal government had little place in mental health. In fact, President Franklin Pierce vetoed an 1854 bill granting federal lands to finance the construction of state mental hospitals, on the grounds that the condition of an individual was none of the federal government's business (Pierce, 1854).

An examination of the history of federal involvement in mental health can enlighten us about the dynamics of the provision of care. It is in the interplay between social and political forces, and professional and scientific developments that we shall find some understanding of how problems come to our attention, how certain solutions seem to emerge, how laws are written, and how new problems are created. Looking at issues with the clarity of vision afforded by hindsight, we shall see that massive social problems create human casualties. Typically, government reacts to the issue by supporting the development of solutions directed to the care of individuals, solutions which tend to obscure the social causes of the human misery that services are meant to mitigate.

Clifford Beers and the organization of a mental health lobby. It is axiomatic that for government to act in relation to a social problem, the problem has to come to public attention, and organized constituencies interested in seeing the problem solved have to act. Clifford Beers, his book, and his organization did not directly influence the federal government until after the Second World War. However, due to his efforts fifty years earlier, a national lobbying organization was in place ready to exert influence when the time came.

In 1900, at the age of 34, Clifford Beers underwent a psychotic episode and was hospitalized for about three years, then discharged. He had a relapse and was rehospitalized. During the latter part of his hospitalization, apparently in a maniclike state, he formulated plans to improve the care of the mentally ill. Keeping careful notes of his experiences and his maltreatment by attendants and physicians, upon his release he wrote *A Mind That Found Itself* (Beers, 1908) hoping to have the same impact on the nation that Harriet Beecher Stowe's book *Uncle Tom's Cabin* had had in an earlier time.

A Mind that Found Itself is a remarkable book as a first-person account of a mental illness. Beers was fortunate in attracting the assistance of William James, who wrote an introduction, and Adolph Meyer, the leading psychiatrist of his day. Although Beers was originally interested in stimulating public sentiment against the mental hospitals, Adolph Meyer influenced him to work toward establishing an organization which would not only have as its mission improving conditions in the hospital, but which would also serve as a permanent agency for reform, public education, and eventually the prevention of mental illness.

Beers, an energetic, charming, manic promoter, organized the Connecticut Society for Mental Hygiene in 1908 and a National Committee for Mental Hygiene by 1909. The National Committee initially directed its efforts toward the reform of mental hospitals, the improvement of facilities for the care of the mentally ill, and improved understanding of the problem (Winters et al., 1969). After World War I, it turned its attention to the development of preventive services and was instrumental in the development of the modern child guidance clinic (Levine & Levine, 1970).

The National Committee for Mental Hygiene merged in 1950 with the Psychiatric Foundation of the American Psychiatric Association and the National Mental Health Foundation to become the National Association for Mental Health. These associations, never as influential as some of the better known health foundations, nonetheless existed as an organized lobby for mental health services. By then, the organization had active chapters in every state and in many local communities. After World War II, the National Association was effective in creating political support at both the state and national levels.

World War I. War is a cataclysmic event in the life of any nation, having profound impact on many aspects of society. The First World War, now dwarfed in our memory by other more recent traumas to our national consciousness, was no different. The nation's need for soldiers required a draft, the Selective Service Act of 1917. The mental fitness of draftees, and the necessity to place men into appropriate positions within the service, led to the development of group intelligence tests and group tests of personality. The first of the personality inventories, the Woodworth Personal Data Sheet, was developed during the war to serve military medical and personnel purposes. The war resulted in a large number of neuropsychiatric casualties, and the care and treatment of the shell-shocked veteran was a matter of grave public concern. After the war, the large number of returning veterans required trained personnel to serve them. The profession of psychiatric social work was created partly to serve that need (Levine & Levine, 1970). The First World War put the federal Veterans Administration in the business of treating mental illness. The war was the occasion for establishing an important precedent for the provision of mental health services by an agency of the federal government, although the Veterans Administration as such did not come into being until 1930 (Fleming, 1957).

Although the war itself was a proximal cause of a mental illness epidemic, there was very little serious professional attention to the prevention of war as a means of preventing neuropsychiatric casualties. The pacifist movement active prior to our entrance into the war was suppressed by the patriotic fervor of the war period, and later by the postwar emphasis on 100 percent Americanism. The postwar conservative political climate supported a turning inward and an emphasis on the problems of individuals (Levine & Levine, 1970).

Prior to World War I, there had been some cooperation between psychiatrists and social workers in developing after care programs. Adolf Meyer was particularly active in that work. Psychopathic hospitals designed to treat acutely disturbed patients close to home developed in the early 1900s (Southard & Jarrett, 1922; Reisman, 1976).

A more than rudimentary social psychiatry developed in the military during the First World War, but that experience had little influence on psychiatry in the 1920s beyond stimulating the growth of professional psychiatric social work (Deutsch, 1949; Levine & Levine, 1970). Psychiatry sought the physical causes of mental disorders. The political climate was unfavorable for a social psychiatric approach because the bulk of those who contributed to the hospital population came from the poor and the foreign born. Concern with social justice and social reform was at low ebb in the 1920s. In fact the term social psychiatry, first used in 1917 by E. E. Southard, founder of a pioneering outpatient clinic at the Boston Psychopathic Hospital, disappeared from use after 1925, not to reappear in an index of a volume of the American Journal of Psychiatry until 1939 (Bell & Spiegel, 1966). Grudging public support could be obtained for the care of those who were ill, but there was no inclination on the part of government to pursue the argument that the conditions of social life were implicated in the mental and emotional difficulties of individuals.

The influence of the Second World War and its immediate aftermath will be considered below. For now, it is sufficient to note that the Veterans Administration was in place and ready to expand to meet the needs of returning veterans. After the Second World War, Veterans Administration training programs were critical for the mental health field. A crash program supported graduate training, internships, and residencies in psychology, social work, and psychiatry. New clinics and hospitals were built, often adjacent to universities or medical centers, with many attractive jobs. In the immediate postwar period, the Veterans Administration mission to care for the returning veteran dominated mental health efforts. Because so much was concentrated on the returning veteran, largely young and middle-aged males, the development of programs for care and for training of personnel to service other populations (e.g., women, children, the aged) was neglected. The emphasis on the returning veteran led to a whole generation of mental health workers without training or encouragement to service other populations. It was the war and its requirements that defined the mental health problem, and defined the solutions the federal government was willing and able to support.

Immigration and mental disorder. Massive immigration prior to the First World War was another social factor leading to federal involvement in mental health services. While today we celebrate our varied ethnic heritages, poor and unwashed immigrants were not always welcomed with open arms, nor did they find a land of milk and honey with streets paved with gold. Not only was life hard, but many Americans were opposed to immigration, believing that only the poorest of foreign stock came here. Henry Goddard tested immigrants at the docks and concluded that 50 percent were feebleminded (Sarason & Doris, 1969).

Studies conducted in New York State in the first quarter of the century showed a higher prevalence of foreign born than native born among those admitted to New York State hospitals. As part of the reaction against immigrants, and related to the rationale for increasingly restrictive legislation, the United States Public Health

Service was given the job of examining and certifying aliens who came to the United States (Brand, 1965; Felix, 1967). Public health efforts were directed toward screening out undesirable immigrants, and not toward an examination of the conditions of life that might have led to their distress and to their apparently high rates of hospitalization for mental illness. The commitment of public resources to the solution of a mental health problem led away from an examination of the conditions of social life.

Narcotics control. The Harrison Narcotics Act of 1914 created another situation leading to the entry of the federal government into mental health services. It is difficult to say how much of a problem narcotics addiction was in the years prior to 1914. There is not much mention of it in the social problems literature produced by progressive era social reformers. Alcoholism was of much greater concern. The introduction of morphine and hypodermic needles during the Civil War created some addicts. Introduced into the United States by the Chinese, opium smoking became something of a general fad. Americans used cocaine and heroin in patent medicines sold over the counter. Legislative prohibitions against narcotics seemed to be related to the impending war. Anything interfering with efficiency was viewed as a great evil. For a while, addicts could receive drugs by prescription from their physicians, but later, perhaps correlated with the prohibition mentality, the availability of drugs for comfort or pleasure was absolutely restricted. No one knows how many people used drugs, but it is estimated the act itself created 100,000 new criminals, now legally cut off from their sources (Musto, 1973).

The problem of the addict was not foreseen when the law was passed, but even the earliest examination of drug usage revealed complex connections between personal and social factors. Addiction could not be dealt with as a problem of law enforcement alone. In 1929, Congress authorized the establishment of two narcotics farms to treat addicts, and a Division of Mental Hygiene within the Public Health Service to oversee the treatment facilities. The first hospital, the famous facility at Lexington, Kentucky, opened in 1935. The passage of the law and its sequaelae was another step putting the federal government into the business of providing mental health services. Once again a massive social problem, this time in part created by federal legislation, resulted in an individually oriented solution. Once again, a social problem was treated as a psychological problem.

Prohibition and its consequences. Alcoholism, a major mental health problem today, was also an important problem in pre-World War I days. The Great Experiment—Prohibition—indirectly created another demand for the provision of mental health services by the federal government. The reasons for prohibition are debatable. One writer has interpreted it as part of the struggle between the older Protestant virtues and the newer eastern European immigrant cultures, a last ditch effort to preserve the values of small town America against change (Gusfield, 1963).

The solution to the saloon problem was one rationale behind prohibition. Workmen were enticed into saloons where they quickly spent their wages on drink, leaving their families hungry. And indeed saloons were a serious problem. There was one for every three hundred of population in some cities. Saloons were unregulated. Authorities claim that saloon keepers, working with liquor and beer manufacturers, enticed workmen to drink and exposed them to crime and vice. Saloons were important gathering places and recreational centers, but they took men away from their families. Social reformers believed that saloons contributed to poverty, crime, vice, personal degredation, and family problems.

In the first few years after the Prohibition Amendment was passed in 1919, there is some evidence that it reduced the incidence of alcoholism as reflected in a declining rate of diagnosis of alcoholic psychosis and in deaths due to cirrhosis of the liver. Prohibition was successful in controlling drinking among the working classes. It was more difficult to produce and transport more bulky products, the beer and wine which workingmen drank. The speakeasy was a middle-class invention. Social workers, who testified to the Wickersham Commission investigating repeal, were unanimous in saying that they rarely saw family problems associated with alcoholism during prohibition (Sinclair, 1964).

While movies emphasize gangsterism and corruption, popular culture underestimates the amount of law enforcement during prohibition. There were five federal prisons and penitentiaries in

1916, housing about 5000 prisoners. In 1929, there were still only five, but these institutions, built to house a maximum of 7000 prisoners, now held 12,000, more than 4000 sentenced for violating the liquor laws. Prison conditions continued to be poor into the 1930s (Sinclair, 1964). Those late-night Pat O'Brien-James Cagney prison films depicting prison riots in the 1930s reflected fact.

The Public Health Service was given the job of providing mental health services to federal prisoners who were rioting partly because, after 1933, they were being held in overcrowded quarters for acts which were no longer crimes. The federal commitment in mental health was once more enlarged (Felix, 1967). Once again, a complex of problems with origins in the social order led to a mental health solution focused on individual problems.

POST-WORLD WAR II

Mental health problems during the war. Information had been available for years that mental health was a prominent problem in American life. Rates per 100,000 of population of patients in mental hospitals had risen from 183.6 in 1904 to 412.6 by 1950. There were 68.2 per 100,000 new admissions to mental hospitals in 1922, and 102.5 per 100,000 by 1950. The reasons for the increase were complex. Goldhamer and Marshall (1953) analyzing admissions to the Worcester State Hospital over a 100-year period concluded that rates of hospitalization had not changed if one took into account population growth and the aging of the population. To some extent increased use reflected an increased number of facilities and greater sophistication about mental health problems. Nevertheless, data showing that mental health was an important problem had been available for years and were well known to epidemiologists. It took the Second World War to draw attention to the problem.

Military data brought the mental health problem to Congressional attention. Draft statistics showed that twelve of every hundred men examined for induction into service were rejected for neuropsychiatric reasons. Of all those rejected by the draft for any reason, 39 percent had a neuropsychiatric diagnosis. Thirty-seven percent of all those discharged from service for disability had neuropsychiatric diagnoses. Considering the men who were rejected for service were in the prime of life, ranging in age from 18 to 37, serious questions were raised about the magnitude of the mental health problem (Felix, 1967).

State hospitals become political liabilities. State hospitals had been thoroughly neglected during the depression and during the war years. After the war, publicity about the scandalous conditions of the state hospitals created a climate conducive to reform. During the war, manpower shortages aggravated poor conditions. In one city, vagrants were given the choice of working in the state hospital or going to jail. In an effort to relieve the personnel shortage, conscientious objectors were assigned to work in some of these institutions. These articulate, sensitive, committed individuals began to call attention to horrible conditions (Brand, 1965).

Albert Deutsch wrote a series of exposés, saying the mental hospitals rivalled "the horrors of the Nazi concentration camps . . . hundreds of naked mental patients herded into huge, barnlike, filth infested wards, in all degrees of deterioration, untended, and untreated, stripped of every vestige of human decency, many in stages of semi-starvation." His stories, which first appeared in 1946 in the short-lived radical newspaper PM were later published in his widely read book *Shame of the States* (Deutsch, 1948). Other books also made their way to the public. A best-selling novel, *The Snake Pit*, and a film based on it aroused popular support. *Life Magazine* ran a story on the Philadelphia State Hospital and *Reader's Digest* condensed O'Gorman's book *Oklahoma Attacks its Snake Pits* in 1948. The widespread publicity not only created a climate of sympathy, but the scandalous conditions made the state hospitals political liabilities for incumbent governors (O'Gorman, 1956).

The Governor's Conference of 1949 sponsored a study of mental health programs in the forty-eight states. The National Association of Mental Health, the direct lineal descendant of Clifford Beer's National Committee of Mental Hygiene, worked to create political support for massive federal efforts in mental health. O'Gorman, by then Executive Director of the National Association for Mental Health, worked with allies among the governors to keep mental health issues alive at state levels. By 1954, a National Governor's Conference on Mental Health was held. The conference supported increased appropriations for hospitals, for training, for research, for community based programs to reduce utilization rates of state hospitals, and for community education (O'Gorman, 1956).

Renewed therapeutic optimism. In the 1860s the psychiatrist Pliny Earle pronounced mental illness incurable. Later, in the 1880s, Emil Kraeplin, who developed the concept of dementia praecox, said the disease was incurable. After that, relatively few mental patients were discharged. While some dissenting voices (e.g., Bleuler, 1950) raised questions about the contribution of conditions of hospitalization to the character of the illness, the dominant psychiatric view was of an illness with an inexorable course. By the 1930s, discharge rates dropped to somewhere between 5 and 20 percent (Bockoven, 1972). Mental illness was a discouraging affair, and mental hospitals, set in isolated areas, had fearsome reputations.

Then, as a consequence of experience in the military, psychiatric viewpoints about mental illness changed drastically. Military experience revealed that psychiatric knowledge and personnel size were completely inadequate to meet the need. Diagnostic skills, so important in state hospital psychiatry, proved all but useless in the military context. State hospital custodial procedures were inappropriate, and the few psychoanalytically trained practitioners knew little of normal development or of cultural variation in behavior and attitude. The psychiatry of the day provided little basis for understanding behavior of men in groups, or for dealing with the variety of personalities and behavior patterns that emerged as disciplinary problems. The futility of diagnosis, and the repeated failure of psychiatric prediction uncovered the inadequacies of existing knowledge to deal with the full range of human problems referred to the mental health worker.

Many men developed disorders during combat, but many others were involuntary recruits having difficulty in adjusting to military life. Civilians not only had to adjust to the military status hierarchy and to impersonal authority and rigid discipline, but also to new social conditions, away from accustomed social roles and away from normal social controls. The high frequency of adjustment problems opened a whole new world to members of the mental health fields, whose horizons had been limited in the past (Stouffer, Suchman, DeVinney, Star, & Williams, 1949).

Wartime exigencies led to therapeutic experimentation. Discoveries concerning the prevention and treatment of combat related conditions, known since the First World War, were rediscovered and extended. Rapid treatment and early return to combat was effective in treating men under stress, presaging the concept of early treatment with minimal disruption in normal roles which was to mark community mental health practice. Intensive therapy, begun early with nurses, psychologists, and social workers as therapists, resulted in the discharge with the diagnosis of "improved" for seven of every ten patients with psychotic diagnoses (Menninger, 1946). Compared to the low rates of discharge from custodial state hospitals, the impressive rates of improvement aroused hopes that civilian mental health problems would also yield to improved treatment. Zusman (1967) states that in civilian hospitals that adopted intensive treatment methods, even before the introduction of psychotropic drugs, ward ambience and the very physical appearance of patients improved.

Postwar optimism. The Second World War ended leaving in its wake a national sense of optimism. Those who grew up with the Viet Nam war, or who have suffered our national sense of helplessness in dealing with foreign and domestic problems, will have difficulty in appreciating the unity of purpose engendered by the war effort. An exceedingly small percentage of soldiers felt the war was meaningless (Stouffer, Lumsdaine, Lumsdaine, Williams, Smith, Janis, Star, & Cottrell, 1949). The nation had pulled together and successfully repelled a threat to its well being. Our enemies were unambiguous villains. War time science produced the wonder drugs—the sulfanilimides, penicillin and later streptomycin. Diseases and infections that had been untreatable were now rapidly conquered. It seemed reasonable to believe that any disease could be cured. Most important, the war ended with the explosion of the first atomic bomb. The bomb was produced quickly in a massive scientific and engineering effort. While the bomb's potential for destruction was understood only dimly, the social potential of its powers exploded into our consciousness. The wonders of a science fiction world were at hand.

Science emerged from the war with an extraordinarily successful partnership with government. A wartime Office of Scientific Research and Development had been established under the direction of Vanevar Bush. Its Committee on Medical Research had stimulated many of the advances in military medicine. Even before the war ended, on Pearl Harbor Day of 1944, President Franklin Roosevelt wrote to Bush asking for recommendations for the continuation of the science-government partnership. Roosevelt was concerned with postwar federal support of science, but he was also interested in stimulating the postwar economy (Brand, 1965; England, 1976). Bush's recommendations included proposals for the support of scientific manpower development and for increased support of university based scientific effort. His report referred to the 7,000,000 Americans who were mentally ill, setting the stage for efforts to ameliorate that problem using the tools of science.

A major step. The National Institute of Mental Health. The United States Public Health Service was an established and respected agency, destined to fall heir to the wartime effort in mental health research. In 1944, Dr. Thomas Parran, the Director of the USPHS, appointed Dr. Robert Felix to head its Division of Mental Hygiene. That division had originated years ago out of the need to screen immigrants, treat drug addicts, and provide psychiatric services to federal prisons, overcrowded with those who had violated the prohibition laws.

Felix, a highly respected psychiatrist, a masterful politician, and a beloved figure to those who worked with him, drafted a far reaching program in mental health. Since no existing law was broad enough to encompass the program, he and Parran worked for a bill for a National Institute of Mental Health. Felix worked hard to win lay, professional, and political support. He wrote to all of the state societies for mental health, the descendants of Clifford Beers' National Committee for Mental Hygiene. He solicited support from the editors of major mental health journals, and invited leading figures in psychiatry, public health, and related fields to testify to Congress. General Lewis B. Hershey, then

Director of the Draft, testified emphasizing the overwhelming rate of rejection from the draft for neuropsychiatric reasons. Military and naval psychiatrists lent their support as well.

The National Mental Health Act passed overwhelmingly, and was signed into law by President Harry S. Truman on July 3, 1946. The Act gave the USPHS broad authority to combat mental illness and to promote mental health. It was empowered to support training, research and demonstration projects, and research in universities, medical schools and research institutes. While waiting for the first appropriation, Felix developed a broad based National Advisory Mental Health Council, including lay and professional leaders. Eventually that advisory body played an important role in the National Institute of Mental Health which was finally established in 1949. Its first appropriation in 1948 was for $4,500,000, but by 1980, its successor agency, the Alcohol, Drug Abuse and Mental Health Administration (ADAMHA) received well over 1 billion dollars (Brand, 1965; Felix, 1967; Foley, 1975).

NIMH's basic policies were formulated and carried through by its professional leadership, working cooperatively with Congress. While the professional and political leadership formulated general policies, implementation of policy relied heavily on professionals outside of government. Most research money went to scientists in the field who initiated proposals for the work they wished to do. Their proposals were reviewed by other non-government scientists who rated them for scientific merit. Committees of non-government scientists advised about promising directions for development. NIMH's National Advisory Council, composed of laymen and non-government scientists, allocated funds generally according to the merit ratings assigned by the peer groups. However, the Council, by law, had to approve awards before NIMH administrators could make them. NIMH professionals also had the benefit of the advice of informed people outside of government who could influence NIMH policies.

The peer review and Advisory Council system was important in generating widespread support of NIMH in the professions and among informed laymen. Throughout its years of operation, the system was free of charges of corruption or of undue political influence. Because of its high degree of professionalism, and the widespread support its policies and practices generated, NIMH moved forward rapidly in its mission of stimulating training, research, and service programs.[1] (See Wildavsky, 1964, for an analysis of bureaucratic budget policies that build constituent support.)

NIMH showed rapid, substantial progress in increasing the number of mental health workers. Training programs, internships, residencies, and fellowships supported large numbers of students in all mental health disciplines in clinical and in research training. Outpatient facilities expanded rapidly (Connery et al., 1968). NIMH was effectively implementing policies supported by state governments and by the federal government when it acted to increase the supply of trained clinicians and research workers.

Progress was made in understanding the biochemistry of stress and stress products. Selye (1946) described the general adaptation syndrome in which prolonged stress led to a breakdown in the chemical defenses of the body, with resulting illness. These advances made real the concept of mental illness as a medical, physiological, organic problem that could respond to physiological treatment. Progress in research, expanding facilities, and growing numbers of trained personnel provided the evidence that further support would continue to be repaid with further advances.

Psychoactive drugs. New drugs with important psychological effects appeared in the early 1950s. One of these was Rauwolfia, or reserpine, an ancient Indian drug whose medicinal properties had been described twenty years earlier. It received scientific

1. The peer review system had until lately been free of criticism. In recent years, however, some critics argued the system stifled creativity, and that it created a power elite with advantages over others in the field who did not participate. Others who have studied its operation claim it is relatively good (Gustafson, 1975). The development of a contract system in contrast to a system of grants for supporting government research, and the government's emphasis on supporting work primarily in its priority areas, may eventually have serious repercussions for scientific freedom, integrity, and vitality. Favoritism—contractors currying favor by producing research results that government officials want—and the lack of opportunity for independent replication and criticism before findings are accepted are all dishearteningly real possibilities that may eventually undercut public confidence in government supported science.

attention because it was useful in reducing blood pressure. It also had a sedative effect, reducing tension and anxiety without inducing stupor. The cautious professional response was amplified by attention in the mass media. Another new drug, chlorpromazine, had been developed in France in the early 1950s. Smith, Klein, and French obtained an exclusive license to market the drug in the United States under the name of Thorazine. SKF encouraged its use in the treatment of mental disorders. The discovery of drugs with psychoactive properties stimulated a vast amount of research and the hopes that much more would be learned about psychopharmacology, and indeed about the biochemistry of the brain itself (Cole & Gerard, 1959).

Although some authorities (e.g., Zusman, 1967) claim that therapeutic optimism predated the widespread use of psychoactive drugs, and that hospital censuses had started to decline before their introduction, drugs stimulated active treatment programs. The drugs did not cure, but they did reduce the most distressing symptoms. Wards could be unlocked and patients discharged. Moreover, drugs could be produced and administered on a mass basis. Within a relatively few years, research resulted in the production of a variety of medications with effectiveness in schizophrenia and depression. The use of minor tranquilizers proliferated. By 1970, tranquilizers accounted for 17 percent of all prescriptions filled in American drug stores (Parry et al., 1973).

In 1955, patients in state and county mental hospitals numbered 559,000. By 1975, that number had declined to 215,000. Admissions and readmissions climbed, and then levelled off (Witkin, 1979). The use of drugs permitted the reduction of hospital censuses and shorter stays on each admission, but if patients were to be maintained in the community, after care, outpatient, and rehabilitative services had to be provided (Kaplan & Bohr, 1976). Because we now had drugs that effectively controlled symptoms, we needed community based services more than ever before.

The Joint Commission on Mental Health and Illness. The Mental Health Study Act of 1955 was a major step toward change. By 1955, a working coalition had formed. It consisted of the professional leadership of NIMH, the leadership of the psychiatric profession, the universities and medical schools receiving training and research support, lobbying organizations such as the National Association of Mental Health with its professional organizers and influential lay persons, and several congressmen and senators who had made medical care and the development of our scientific resources their special concern. Each year, NIMH was able to go back to Congress with a strong appeal for increased funds, based on a record of performance and with formidable support from the Governors of each state, and from the professions (Connery et al., 1968; Foley, 1975).

In 1953, the American Medical Association and the American Psychiatric Association held a joint conference on mental health. The conference called for a National Report to set standards for the future (O'Gorman, 1956). Given the favorable climate of opinion and political support, it was timely. NIMH had carried out its tasks with competence and with broad professional support. An effective treatment for an age-old problem seemed to be at hand, and it was in keeping with the spirit of faith in science and technology to conquer all. In February 1955, Congress unanimously passed a resolution to provide for "an objective, thorough, and nationwide analysis and reevaluation of the human and economic problems of mental illness."

The study was conducted by the Joint Commission on Mental Health and Illness, a private nonprofit corporation, an outgrowth of a planning body initiated by the American Medical Association and the American Psychiatric Association and financed in part by Smith, Kline, and French. The Joint Commission's trustees consisted of representatives of the AMA, the American Psychiatric Association, the American Psychological Association, the American Association of Psychiatric Social Workers, the American Hospital Association, the American Nursing Association, the National League of Nursing, and the National Education Association. The Commission itself was composed of 36 representatives of lay and professional agencies and organizations covering a wide spectrum of interests. The American Legion, for example, provided funds which supported distribution of the Joint Commission's final report (Foley, 1975).

The Joint Commission had excellent professional leadership. It produced a number of important reports, including its summary volume *Action for Mental Health* (1961). Jahoda's *Current*

Concepts of Positive Mental Health (1958), Albee's *Mental Health Manpower Trends* (1959), and Veroff, Feld, and Gurin's *Americans View Their Mental Health. A National Survey.* (1960) were extremely influential in shaping views of the mental health problem. The other reports were also highly competent, but more specialized, and so less obviously influential.

The Joint Commission's final report was, in many respects, a forward-looking document. It urged continued support for professional education and for research. Recognizing the importance of Albee's cogent statement of the limitations on training sufficient professional personnel to meet service needs, it endorsed the use of a variety of nonmedical personnel in treatment roles, and it supported the development of outpatient care to prevent hospitalization. Recognizing that most people took their troubles to caregivers other than trained mental health professionals, it endorsed education and consultation programs with front line workers (clergy, family physicians, teachers, probation workers, public health nurses, judges, welfare workers, police).

At the same time, however, the report's essential thrust was the recommendation to revitalize the state hospital system. The Joint Commission proposed limiting the size of institutions to prevent the worst abuses of custodial care. Despite its recognition of the need for extensive services on an outpatient basis to many people in need, and despite its recognition of the necessity for preventive services, it emphasized that the central mental health problem was the care of the severely mentally ill.

The Joint Commission's report has been severely criticized for emphasizing inpatient care at the expense of prevention. Figures clearly show the overall magnitude of the mental health problem; for example, Albee's (1959) analysis that there would never be enough professionally trained mental health personnel to provide treatment to all who needed it. Norman Polansky, a member of two of the Joint Commission's committees, responded to criticism with the comment: "It was not so simple. One could choose between annointing the Camp Fire Girls as an agency of positive mental health, or confronting the Eisenhower administration with the stench of our state hospitals" (Polansky, 1971, p. 211).

Polansky's comment not only reveals the necessarily political orientation of those who consider national policy, but it also reveals the conflict that members of the Joint Commission must have experienced in developing its recommendations. In his introduction to the Joint Commission's report, Executive Director Dr. Jack Ewalt gave some hint that the Joint Commission's report was necessarily a compromise of a variety of interests, as might be expected from the broad-based composition of the Joint Commission's membership. Some were in favor of fundamentally restructuring the system of care; others believed that care of the seriously mentally ill was the fundamental responsibility, and that the state hospital would continue to be the cornerstone of that system of care.

Ewalt pointed out that recommendations which did not command a unanimity of professional support would leave Congress with the option of taking no action, on the grounds that if the professionals could not agree, there was no clearly supportable course of action. The Joint Commission's recommendations seemed to have been shaped by what was politically sound. The recommendations were not dictated solely by the data, but rather varied professional interests had to be recognized and supported, and the probable viewpoint of professional politicians and legislators had to be kept in mind.

Given the complexity within which the system of care operates, such political compromise is inevitable. As long as funds for care derive from the body politic, and as long as we recognize that there are disparate professional, power, economic, and status issues involved in the system of service delivery, it is necessary to examine the influence of such factors to understand our system of care.

SUMMARY

Our review of the early history of federal involvement in mental health has taken us along a winding path. Events of national significance—war, immigration, narcotics control, prohibition—had correlates in human problems. As the human problems came to political awareness, solutions emerged. Often the solutions were piecemeal, and directed toward the treatment of individuals in distress. This was necessary, of course, but the focus on individuals obscured consideration of the social origins of the problem.

It is also true that past is prologue, in the sense that past actions set the stage for future actions. Once a state hospital system existed, it was no longer possible to wipe it out and start from scratch when it proved inadequate to its task. Clifford Beers' crusade to reform the mental hospital left an organization that provided political support for a national program of a scope never envisioned by Beers. The several halting steps toward mental health service delivery by the Public Health Service fathered a Division of Mental Hygiene, an agency which was ready and willing to take advantage of the opportunity to develop a comprehensive mental health program that arose after the war. After World War II, political support for improved mental health care, scientific developments, and economic policy to stimulate economic growth by fostering education and science, converged to produce funds for mental health on a grander scale. The initial steps creating broad-based support for mental health activities also created a constituency whose interests had to be taken into account. Later, as we shall see, all the professionals who were trained with NIMH funds also became a constituency, albeit a diverse one, for the continuation of federal support.

Each step was informed by some data, but in the final analysis what emerged was as much a product of what was possible in a political sense as it was the most desirable option from either a scientific or a clinical viewpoint. We shall see similar processes when we examine the implementation of President Kennedy's comprehensive community mental health program in the next chapter.

Chapter 3

THE COMMUNITY MENTAL
HEALTH CENTERS ACT
Implementation in a Political Context

John F. Kennedy took office as the first President born in this century. He was a man of vision and charisma who projected the image of a better future for all. He took office just as the Joint Commission's report was made to the Congress. Kennedy saw the need and the opportunity. He called for a "bold new approach." That approach turned out to be the Community Mental Health Centers Act of 1963 (PL 88-164). How it was implemented is the subject of this chapter.

THE FEDERAL CONTEXT

Kennedy's Message to Congress. The Joint Commission made its report to Congress on December 30, 1960. Kennedy took office a few days later. The Joint Commission's report had earlier influenced a plank in the Democratic platform. It was also endorsed by the 1961 Annual Governor's Conference. Shortly afterwards, President Kennedy appointed a Presidential Task Force, including professional bureaucrats from NIMH and from the Bureau of the Budget, knowledgeable political appointees representing several government interests, and a special assistant to the Secretary of HEW who had direct access to the White House. The Task Force heard testimony from various NIMH officials, from state mental health commissioners, and from other state officials. The Task Force's job was to determine what was politically and economically feasible, and scientifically reasonable. The

Task Force's report to the President resulted in Kennedy's Message to the Congress on Mental Illness and Mental Retardation (Connery et al., 1968; Foley, 1975).

President Kennedy, who had a personal interest in mental retardation, delivered his Message to the Congress on February 5, 1963. The message marked the first time a President of the United States took specific cognizance of the problems of mental illness and retardation, and stated national policy. Emphasizing the financial cost and the tragedies affecting individuals and families, the President called for a "bold new approach."

Kennedy emphasized the need to develop preventive programs, and in so doing accepted the key concept that environmental conditions were causally related to mental illness and mental retardation.

> Prevention will require both selected specific programs directed especially at known causes, and the general strengthening of our fundamental community, social welfare, and educational programs which can do much to eliminate or correct the harsh environmental conditions which often are associated with mental retardation and mental illness. (Kennedy, 1963, p.2)

The President revealed considerable philosophical kinship with reformers of an earlier day who also saw much of the cause of distress in the conditions of social life (Levine & Levine, 1970). In tying the cause of problems to social issues, Kennedy revealed the commitment to social change that later received expression in his and in President Lyndon Johnson's Great Society programs. His message emphasized the relationship between poverty and retardation:

> The only feasible program with a hope for success must not only aim at the specific causes and control of mental retardation, but seek solutions to the broader problems of our society with which mental retardation is so intimately related. (p.2)

Emphasizing the problems of cultural and educational deprivation, he linked his proposals to the development of federal aid for elementary and secondary education. His message set a tone to explore at a national level a variety of approaches to the provision of assistance to people in need. The convergence of the political and the social with the professional and the scientific is nowhere better exemplified than in Kennedy's message, and in what was to become the new fields of community psychology and community mental health.

Kennedy's message went well beyond the Joint Commission in several respects. Where the Joint Commission emphasized the revitalization of the state hospital, the President set as a goal the halving of the institutionalized population and the establishment of community based treatment.

> If we launch a broad new mental health program now, it will be possible within a decade or two to reduce the number of patients now under custodial care by 50 per cent or more. Many more mentally ill can be helped to remain in their own homes without hardship to themselves or their families. Those who are hospitalized can be restored to useful life. (p.2)

To implement the concept of community based care, Kennedy called for the development of comprehensive community mental health centers, which would have all the services necessary to ensure a continuum of treatment.

> As his needs change, the patient could move without difficulty or delay to different services—from diagnosis to cure to rehabilitation—without need to transfer to different institutions located in different communities. (p.3)

Each center would provide preventive as well as therapeutic services. Provision would be made in each center's program for consultative services, and for mental health information and education.

Federal aid would help establish the centers, but the major proportion of their funds would come from state and local sources, and from health insurance and other third party payments. Kennedy's advisors anticipated that funds would be redirected from institutional to community based care as the institutional population decreased.[1] Many different kinds of organizations were eli-

1. Foley (1975) believes that at that time, Congressional and NIMH leaders were not at all adverse to eventually supporting the centers totally with federal funds. Influential economists (e.g., Galbraith, 1958) were currently arguing that economic growth required greater expediture in the public sector. A spending program for mental health services was in keeping with such economic policy. The decision to require joint federal, state, and local funding reflected the traditions of our federal

gible to sponsor community mental health centers—gen
pitals with psychiatric units, outpatient facilities, state
hospitals, private nonprofit agencies, or consortia of agen

The issues of who could sponsor a community mental
center and how they would be financed are political in nature. A
diversity of sponsorship was congruent with the characteristics of
the existing system of care. And using both local and state funding
agreed with the traditions of our federal system of government.
Both of these factors, the existing service system and its interests,
and the sources of funding and their impact on the types of
services to be delivered, were to have important influence in
determining how the centers developed and functioned. When
the community mental health center was proposed, the federal
legislation seemed to promise a partnership in a new venture.
How that partnership worked out will be pursued further below.
The implementation of Kennedy's new concept was bound to be
affected by the context in which it was implemented.

Planning for Community Mental Health Centers. Kennedy's
Message to the Congress was followed by the Community Mental
Health Centers Act of 1963 (PL 88-164). In deference to political
opposition from the professional leadership of the American
Medical Association, the bill initially omitted funds for staffing,
but authorized the construction of mental health centers (Connery et al., 1968; Foley, 1975).

Each state developed a statewide plan designating catchment
areas, geographic areas serving populations of no less than 75,000
and no more than 200,000, ranked according to their need for
mental health services. The catchment areas took into account
political and geographic boundaries, and were to fit within census
tracts. Planning was to be coordinated with any other ongoing
planning in health, urban redevelopment, or welfare (Surgeon

---

system. It was also grounded in the concept that local financial responsibility
would ensure responsivity to local need. However, had politicians and planners
paid some attention to social history, they would have been aware that local
governments were rarely enthusiastic about paying for welfare or mental hospital
costs (Grob, 1966; Coll, 1969). Some of the centers' financial difficulties following
the end of federal financing could have been anticipated.

General's Ad Hoc Committee on Planning for Mental Health Facilities, 1961).

The catchment area concept was useful in determining the number of centers to be built. It also helped to delineate who would be entitled to care—all those residing within the catchment area boundaries. The requirement was designed to eliminate the possibility that centers would choose to serve select clientele. Any one who lived within the catchment area, and who needed service, must be served. Diagnosis, prognosis, age, sex, race, or ability to pay were not to be barriers to receiving care.[2]

Although the catchment area concept was useful for many purposes, it was not based on any view of a community as an organic entity with its own life and with resources that could be brought to bear in some integrated fashion. The delineation of catchment areas set a direction for services that continues to have important effects. For example, mental health centers in sparsely populated areas cover huge geographic territories in order to encompass a sufficient number of people. Transportation emerged as a major variable to be considered in the provision of effective rural mental health services (Task Panel on Rural Mental Health, 1978). Catchment area boundaries in urban areas sometimes violated natural neighborhood boundaries, necessitating the accommodation of different racial and ethnic groups. In fairness to the architects of the catchment area concept, useful definitions of communities were and still are lacking (Sarason, 1974).

All fifty states submitted planning progress reports by March 1965. Lyndon Johnson, now President, sent his 1965 Health Message to Congress recommending the Medicare program and staffing grants for community mental health centers. The AMA, raising the spectre of socialized medicine, still opposed federal funds for staffs, and Congress worried about whether state and local communities would accept financial responsibility to continue

---

2. Eligibility for care can be a serious problem. I once encountered a child who carried diagnoses of epilepsy, mental retardation, and psychosis. She was shunted from agency to agency with none accepting responsibility. Each specialized agency (e.g., for epilepsy) rejected her claim because of her other diagnoses (i.e., she was psychotic and should be treated by an agency for psychotic children). Apparently, if she accumulated enough diagnoses, she would have been ineligible for all services.

mental health programs after federal funds ceased (Legislative History, PL 89-105). However, Johnson's 1964 election victory was overwhelming and his influence was sufficient to override remaining doubts. The 1965 Act (PL 89-105) providing staffing grants passed readily. The legislation allowed NIMH to bypass state mental health authorities and to deal directly with local sponsors of community mental health centers. This provision created local constituencies for NIMH funded service programs and set the stage for conflict between state authorities and local groups (Foley, 1975).

With the passage of the Community Mental Health Centers Act, and its subsequent extensions, the federal role in mental health services was enlarged considerably. The construction program and the planning efforts of the previous two years had set in motion potent forces. Moreover, mental health care became further involved in the labyrinth of massive government. The ideas and the theory of community mental health had to be implemented through governmental processes. The theory in textbooks and the law in law books are not the same as the theory in practice, nor the law in action.

Early implementation of the 1963 CMHC Act. From the outset, political considerations influenced the implementation of the national policy. Generally speaking, federal funds are distributed so that less wealthy states get more federal money than more affluent states. This policy played a role in decisions about where and how much money was to be distributed once funds were appropriated. Bloom (1977) points out how the formulas, based on population and per capita income, allow poorer states to receive a larger share of federal funds, and to provide fewer local dollars. Regulations also required that new facilities had to be created. The aim of such provisions was to prevent states from shifting the burden of financial costs from the state to the federal government. It may have been that NIMH leaders, sensing that state mental health bureaucracies would be slow in starting Community Mental Health Centers (see Schulberg & Baker, 1975), and wanting to increase their options to move rapidly and show progress to Congress, welcomed the opportunity to deal with many other groups (Foley, 1975).

Local communities vary greatly in their affluence and in the willingness to support services. Nonfederal hard dollars had to be found as matching funds to qualify. Under those circumstances, Bloom (1977) asserts that it was common for communities with the greatest need for mental health services to fail to take advantage of federal funds, while other communities better endowed in dollars and professional resources were able to move rapidly. Taking the long view that eventually all communities would have CMHCs, as originally envisioned, those responsible for implementing the CMHC program were willing to live with the mismatch, on the assumption that it would all be evened out in the end (Foley, 1975).

Such hopes did not reckon with the effects of the Viet Nam war on the American economy, on the ghetto riots, and on the national will to provide services for its citizens. It did not anticipate a new administration with a different philosophy of government and a different view of the responsibility of government to provide health, education, and welfare services. But this was to come later. Let us first examine the local context within which CMHCs were to be developed.

THE LOCAL CONTEXT

The CMHC Act recognized the diversity of services existing in local communities, but it failed to recognize their fragmentation. It also failed to recognize that in order to maintain patients in communities, a range of services not generally included under mental health would be necessary. Housing, income maintenance, transportation, and vocational and recreational needs would have to be met. The CMHC Act was also developed and implemented in isolation from other federal acts (Medicare, Medicaid, Supplemental Security Income) that provided incentives to state governments to deinstitutionalize rapidly. The lack of coordination was to have disasterous consequences in some places.

Who has responsibility? Connery et al. (1968) described a multiplicity of local governmental units (e.g., state, city, county, town, school districts) and private agencies responsible for health, mental health, education, welfare, housing, employment, recreation, and criminal justice. These units have overlapping jurisdictions and responsibilities and compete for tax and philanthropic dollars. Syracuse, New York, a standard metropolitan statistical area with a population of about 620,000 in 1967, had some 228 general and special purpose local authorities, all with interests in some aspects of community life.

The New York State Community Mental Health Services Act of 1954 established the County Mental Health Board as the central body responsible for mental health services. However, mental health authority is separate from other health services, and both are separate from the welfare department. Local, state, and federal agencies do not have exact counterparts, and their geographic districts as well as their bureaucratic structures are uncoordinated. Education and special education are also independent of other service agencies, and to some extent of each other, making it difficult to develop coordinated services for children. The medical school in Syracuse was another independent body with interests in a facility useful for research and training purposes. As Connery et al. put it:

> No one level of government or agency enjoys a monopoly of clinical services, nor is any one category of service totally and exclusively the responsibility of a particular department or bureau. The clinical domain of the local voluntary and private mental illness and retardation services is basically pluralistic in structure and operation and does not present a common front in dealing with the problems raised by mental disorders in the SMSA. Communities seem unable to correct this situation. (p.301)

Such problems in planning persist and are unsolved (Sauber, 1976).

Over and beyond governmental agencies, the private sector exerts an influence on government through the needs of private agencies for funds, and through the efforts of community leaders who serve on boards of local agencies. Community leaders often have a loyal interest in the agency, and they will defend it when under attack or will assist in it seeking funds from public and private sources. Central funding agencies such as the United Way attempt to minimize competition among services by avoiding "duplication of service." Graziano (1969) believes that such a concept protects the local professional power structure against competition from interlopers. Whatever the reason, local service agencies tend to be highly specialized in name, if not in actuality, although they compete for resources and sometimes for clients. Comprehensive and continued care had to be developed in this complex matrix of existing services and vested interests.

In addition to problems that emerge out of the desire of agencies to guard their autonomy, personality conflicts and legal and administrative roadblocks interfere with effective coordination. In some communities, concerns about the invasion of privacy, and problems of public versus private, or local versus state responsibility have added to the heat, if not to the light. It is not infrequent that the local governmental official responsible for mental health care will be at odds with medical school officials, with administrators of state funded programs, or with United Way officials who seek partial governmental funding. In recent years the proliferation of contract agencies and services operated by community groups (e.g., women's collectives, youth groups, racial groups) have added to the competetive atmosphere. Thus it has been difficult to plan consistently or to develop truly cooperative relationships among agencies (Levine, 1980). Given the complexity of the context, it is remarkable that as many centers started as did. It is less remarkable that critics claim that innovative services and continuous care has not developed (Chu & Trotter, 1974). The conditions almost guaranteed that limited progress would be made. Baker and his colleagues (Baker, 1972; Baker, Broskowski, & Brandwein, 1973; Baker, 1974; Baker & Broskowski, 1974; Schulberg & Baker, 1975) have provided excellent analyses of these problems from a systems perspective.

Obtaining services in a fragmented context. The problem of coordinating services in a fragmented context boggle the mind and quickly wear down all but the most hardy. In 1966, we described our experience in working with community agencies:

> [Our] purpose . . . is to serve fair warning to any mental health professional that if he truly becomes involved with the community, he will also become involved, sometimes it seems inextricably, with all the agencies, and all their regulations and attendant bureaucratic structure. The professional should be prepared to

spend long, wearying, frustrating, and only occasionally fruitful hours in telephone conversations, individual meetings and group meetings in order to get some action in a given case. (Sarason et al., 1966)

Examples of the problem abound. It begins with the simple problem of obtaining information about available resources and under what circumstances they may be utilized. Mentally disabled individuals with low and moderate incomes are eligible for HUD assisted housing. HUD had originally defined tenant eligibility based on its definition of a term in the 1959 Housing Act. HUD decided that mentally retarded individuals were not included. In 1971, based on an inquiry from the Michigan State Housing Development Authority, the HUD General Counsel ruled that retarded individuals whose retardation was based on an under-lying physical impairment were eligible. The General Counsel's ruling was not communicated to HUD's Regional and Area offices. A number of months later, HUD issued instructions for imple-menting its subsidized housing project for the handicapped. The instruction continued to define physical handicaps only, and did not refer to the General Counsel's statement to Michigan seven months earlier. Very few Regional Office specialists in housing for the handicapped were aware of the change.

In 1971 and in 1974 presidential directives requested agencies to cooperate with deinstitutionalization programs. In 1976, very few HUD regional and area officials were aware of the directives, much less had they taken action to implement them. At the time of the Comptroller General's study (Comptroller General of the United States, 1977), only one area office could be identified as having taken any sustained action to provide housing for the mentally disabled, and that came about as the result of the initia-tive of a single employee who took the trouble to inquire about available programs.

Consequent to the Comptroller General's report and to the report of the U.S. Senate Subcommittee on Long Term Care (1976), NIMH sponsored a working conference of government agency officials and those who had been working in the commun-ity with long-term care and with community living arrangements for the mentally disabled (NIMH, 1976). The participants were among the most experienced and sophisticated in the nation. Yet at this conference, Jerry Dincin, Executive Director of the Thresholds Psychosocial Rehabilitation Center in Chicago, said in response to a HUD official's statement:

> To me, the most critical thing I have heard this morning is a definitive statement, from the highest echelon in HUD that we could possibly reach, that former psychiatric patients are eligible. This is the first time that I have heard that definitely and absolutely. That means the definition of handicapped *does* include the former psychiatric patient that we are so concerned about. Now we just have to work the system so that we can get him in. (NIMH, 1976, p.58)

It was not just bureaucratic inertia that stood in the way. HUD officials had grave concerns about having mentally handicapped people living in their housing projects, and they believed they could not control the housing agencies which actually owned and operated HUD-assisted housing. Operators of HUD-assisted housing rightly believe the mentally handicapped will need additional assistance, but no funds for such assistance are available. In addition, regulations permit housing authorities to set standards to protect residents from socially disruptive people. From their viewpoint mental patients are trouble, so they have reacted with benign neglect.

Even when services are available, and when agencies are willing to work together, eligibility requirements and the nature of interagency relationships present barriers. Sarason et al. (1966) have described experiences in trying to obtain interagency cooperation to ameliorate the problems that children and families encounter. The following example is typical of the absurd functioning of bureaucracy.

A school consultant had followed a multi-problem family for about two years. Once he attended a conference called by the Visiting Nurses Association (VNA) to develop a plan for assisting Mrs. M. and her large family. Mrs. M. was scheduled for surgery and there was concern about how she would be able to manage her children while she was recovering. In attendance with the VNA nurse and her supervisor was a school nurse and her supervisor, the principal of the school, a school social worker, a welfare worker, and the consulting psychologist working out of a private agency, the Yale Psychoeducational Clinic. The family was renting in a building slated for razing when urban renewal came to that part of the city. Therefore the municipal housing authority and the federal relocation agency was involved. The departments of Pediatrics and Obstetrics of the University Hospital had submitted reports. One child was at a home for delinquent girls and another had just been referred to juvenile court.

The welfare worker was new to her agency, and while there was a thick case file, she had seen the family only once in the previous six months. When asked, she said it would be her legal obligation to pursue any evidence of violation of welfare regulations. Clinical confidentiality could not be invoked at this meeting. Thus the consultant, who knew about a supportive male not living in the home, and who knew about the housework the mother had been doing for additional income, could not share the information.

After nearly two hours of discussion, the welfare worker agreed the mother's laundry allowance could be increased. In view of the woman's precarious state of health (she had been referred for surgery), she was eligible for homemaker services. However, welfare regulations limited the hourly rate for homemakers to $1.25, and since the going rate for household help was well above that amount, the welfare worker doubted that a homemaker could be found, even if funds were available.

Each agency had a thick file, with duplicated information, but all were stymied in providing the most minimal assistance for the family. This example centered on a multi-problem welfare family, but the issues are no different for families with retarded individuals, or for deinstitutionalized mental patients. And it is not as if these problems have newly come to our attention. Warner's classic work *American Charities* was published in 1894, 1908, and 1919. He reported a case in which the worker and supervisor contacted 15 agencies, made 76 visits, wrote 21 letters, and held 41 interviews in the office, all in the days before the telephone. In that instance, the client received some help, according to his report. But the problem is structural. It follows from our creation of many limited-purpose agencies, none of which have the resources or authority to deal with people as if they were whole human beings, not a bundle of needs that can be separated into independently manageable fragments.

Several experiments in coordinating services have been tried and they have failed. Sometimes superficial cooperation was sustained until funding for the experiment ran out, and then it ceased. For example, a common center for all services was opened in one neighborhood. The client brought in by each service was supposed to be served by all the others as well.

It quickly became apparent that cooperation was difficult. Each agency had a different statutory base, had different eligibility requirements, and different reporting requirements. The group was unable to develop a common application. The client had to go from desk to desk filling out separate forms, duplicating information. The agencies had different working hours and regulations; workers responded to different supervisors, and attended meetings at their own agencies, meetings which took workers away from the site but without the knowledge of other agency workers on the site. Personality and jurisdictional conflicts interfered with cooperative action (NIMH, 1976). In general, there were as many barriers to cooperation in a single facility as had existed when they were located separately. This NIMH report is entirely consistent with our own experience in working in a similar cooperative center (Sarason et al., 1966) and with observations about a state and county venture in sharing staff in a common facility (Levine, 1980).

Based on our experience in working in a local community, in 1966 we said:

> It is our belief that the concept of a whole person is violated by the legal division of responsibility for the care of people into pieces that follow arbitrary lines laid down by accidents of history, by a legal rather than a human view of the way people live, and by the exigencies of the political climate that permit one program but not another. However they grew, current practices in many instances do not serve human needs, and urgently require re-evaluation from the point of view of human needs. (Sarason et al., p.269)

There is nothing that we have seen in the interim that has required us to change our minds. Continuity of care was to fight an uphill battle from the very beginning.

THE FEDERAL CONTEXT REVISITED

From 1965 to 1970 the Congress, satisfied with initial progress, continued to renew the Community Mental Health Centers Act and extended it to include services for alcoholics and drug abusers. In 1968 Congress also stipulated that one percent of grant and contract funds appropriated for the Alcohol, Drug Abuse and Mental Health Administration (ADMHA) be allocated to evaluation of the effectiveness and the functioning of the CMHCs. That action stimulated a booming interest in evaluation among research workers in consulting firms and in universities. A new professional specialty developed along with a burgeoning literature. A later law (PL 94-63) allocated 2 percent to evaluation and made it mandatory that every center conduct evaluations. Some of what we know about community mental health centers came from research supported by evaluation funds.

In 1970, acting on recommendations of the Joint Commission on Mental Health of Children (Joint Commission, 1969), Congress authorized increased funds for services for children. At the same time, recognizing that local communities were curtailing services or jettisoning programs as their federal funding expired, Congress extended the staffing grant program. Programs in poverty areas were stimulated by providing additional financial incentives and by easing the requirement to initiate centers with full services as called for in the initial act. Special funds were designated to support consultation and education programs which had so far lagged in development.

By 1967, 186 CMHCs had received federal support, a number that grew to 450 by 1970. From 1970 on the growth rate slowed drastically. By 1973 there were only 493 federally funded CMHCs, and not all of those were fully operational. By 1975, 603 had received some funds, but only 507 were operational.

Congress continued to authorize funds, but from 1970 onward, the Nixon administration expressed its opposition to the CMHC concept and to expenditures for research and training in health and mental health generally. President Nixon impounded funds Congress had authorized and refused to spend them. He lost a court battle on the issue and funds were released (*National Council of CMHCs* v *Weinberger*, 1973).

The following years under Nixon and then under President Ford continued to be lean, in administrative support if not in actual funds. In 1975 Congress overrode President Ford's veto of an act extending and revising the Community Mental Health Centers Act. Additional funds were authorized for mandatory services for children and the elderly. Consultation and education services were extended. Attributable to the activities of the women's movement (Brownmiller, 1975), the Act provided treatment and prevention services for rape victims. Collaboration among community agencies was required. Services consistent with cultural, linguistic, and socioeconomic considerations were required as well. Increased citizen participation in policy formation was mandated. A system of program monitoring and confidential record keeping was specified. The 1975 action in overriding a presidential veto clearly indicated Congressional intent to support CMHCs nationally (Legislative History, PL 94-63; see also Bloom, 1977, for an excellent summary of CMHC legislation over the years).

Since Congress passed a law, it must be so. The Community Mental Health Centers Amendments of 1975 reads in part as follows:

Sec. 302. (a) The Congress finds that—

(1) community mental health care is the most effective and humane form of care for a majority of mentally ill individuals;

(2) the federally funded community mental health centers have had a major impact on the improvement of mental health care by—

(A) fostering coordination and cooperation between various agencies responsible for mental health care which in turn has resulted in a decrease in overlapping and more efficient utilization of available resources;

(B) bringing comprehensive community mental health care to all in need within a specific geographic area regardless of ability to pay; and

(C) developing a system of care which insures continuity of care for all patients, and thus are a national resource to which all Americans should enjoy access. (Title III, Sec. 302, PL 94-63)

Is Congressional optimism warranted by available research? Table 16 in the Legislative History accompanying PL 94-63 shows the reduction in the patient population of state and county mental hospitals. Table 17 provides data from 94 of the 294 centers operating in 1971. The table is titled "Statistics Bearing on CMHC Program Objectives: Decrease in Inappropriate Utilization of State Hospitals." The data are interpreted as showing that as CMHCs mature (are in operation more than 3 years), rates of hospitalization and rates of admission to state and county mental hospitals decrease. These are the only data reported in the Legislative History. It is in the nature of the advocacy approach of the law that no counterinterpretations and no data contrary to that position are presented or discussed. We have already seen that the congressional view of coordination and cooperation, and of continuity of care is probably overly optimistic. What do the data actually say?

While there is good evidence that community mental health practice may accomplish some of its aims (see below), there are alternative interpretations to the one that good patient care is responsible for the decline. If it is a defect of politicians and lawyers that they look at one side of a problem, it is a defect of social researchers to be overly impressed with numbers, and not to look past them to their human meanings. Few of the studies explored policies of admission and discharge pursued by hospitals in areas with and without CMHCs, and assumed uncritically that a reduction in the state hospital population was an absolute good.

We need to examine other variables and other sources of data if we are to conclude that the decline in the state hospital population is indeed a victory for community mental health theory. In some instances community mental health rhetoric may well have served as a convenient rationalization for policies and practices based on far less noble considerations.

FINANCIAL INCENTIVES AND COMMUNITY BASED CARE

"We are hung up, then, on categories of people, services and preferential matching rates, and we have a kind of gamesmanship going around—you could call it a shell game, if you want to

think of it that way." (Emily Nichols, Chief, Health Services
Branch, Medical Assistance Administration, HEW.) (NIMH, 1976,
p.66)

A potent incentive to states to reduce hospital censuses were
laws providing financial means for states to reduce the burdens
on their budgets while shifting the burden to the federal level.
The laws providing financial incentives for emptying the state
hospitals are critical, and it is to these laws and their effects that
we now turn.

Medicare. In 1965 President Lyndon Johnson asked the Congress to provide "the best health care for all Americans regardless
of age, geography or economic status." The Medicare and Medicaid programs were passed in that year. That Act, and later
amendments and revisions, had profound effects on mental health
care, first of the aged, and then on other patients.

Medicare is a form of health insurance designed to pay hospital
and related costs for those over 65 years of age who have social
security benefits, and for those who have received social security
disability benefits for two years. Part A of Medicare covers
inpatient care. Part B covers physicians' charges and other medical services. In general, Medicare works very effectively in covering in-hospital costs for general medical and surgical care.

Medicare is considerably less effective in providing for psychiatric care. There is a lifetime limit of 190 days of in-hospital
coverage if a patient is hospitalized in a psychiatric hospital. The
lifetime limit does not apply to patients treated psychiatrically in
a general hospital, where benefits are the same for mentally ill
patients as they are for all other patients. The financing structure
encourages the use of general physician services not designed for
the treatment of mental illness (Task Panel on Costs and Financing, 1978).

Part B of Medicare provides reimbursement of physician
charges if treated in an inpatient or outpatient facility. However,
if a patient is not hospitalized, but is treated psychiatrically as an
outpatient in the doctor's office, in the patient's own home, or in a
nursing home, then reimbursement cannot exceed 50 percent of
treatment expenses, or $250, whichever is less. That amount of
money covers but a handful of visits at current psychiatric rates,

and is totally insufficient for chronic patients. Thus Medicare reimbursement rules place a premium on hospitalizing patients in general care facilities, because those services are reimbursed by the federal government. Medicare makes it relatively difficult to obtain long-term outpatient care for psychiatric disorders.

Medicare rules promote the revolving door for hospitalization in a general hospital. The number of in-hospital days covered by Medicare in any single spell of illness is limited. However, a spell of illness ends and a new benefit period begins when one is out of the hospital for sixty days and not receiving skilled nursing care in some other setting (Social Security Act, Title XVIII, Sec. 1861). The patient is then entitled to full hospital benefits for a new spell of illness (Sec. 1812). Figures showing reductions in hospitalization are for patients in state and county mental hospitals. They do not include admissions to other facilities reimbursable by the federal government. If, for example, a mature CMHC developed a working relationship with a general hospital, and used that facility for inpatient care of Medicare eligible patients, they would not show up on counts of patients in state and county mental hospitals, although hospitalized. Theoretically, a general hospital working with a CMHC could discharge a Medicare-eligible patient when the end of the patient's paid days approached, keep the patient from being readmitted for 60 days, then readmit and start the cycle all over again.

The theory is not fanciful. Bass (1973) points out that as CMHCs mature, and their staffing grants decline, a greater proportion of their income comes from third-party reimbursements. Landsberg and Hammer (1977) found that recidivists accounted for two thirds of all in-hospital admissions and three fourths of all inpatient days. The authors state:

> The net result of this health insurance scheme is that the inpatient unit of a community mental health center serves as the key element as regards the ability to generate fee income. In the authors' investigation it was found that the inpatient unit of a center often generated up to two-thirds or more of the fee income. It must further be indicated that in order to maximize income, then, inpatient utilization must be maintained at a high level (especially of patients who have insurance coverage). In the simplest terms, it means that "beds must be kept filled." (Landsberg & Hammer, 1977, p.65)

Medicare is based on a medical model, no matter how inappropriate for the care of mental patients. Medicare sets standards for hospitals eligible to provide mental health services under its programs, and also for the Medicaid program (see below). To receive Medicare reimbursement for mental health services, a hospital must be accredited by the Joint Commission on Accreditation of Hospitals or meet equivalent requirements. Medicare also imposes staffing requirements for inpatient care, including staff for psychiatric, medical, surgical, nursing, social work, psychological, and activities therapies. The regulations support care in a hospital geared for acute intensive treatment in the classical medical model, but make no provision for care in alternative facilities more suitable for chronic patients.

Medicare regulations require that discharge summaries and aftercare or follow-up plans be included in medical records. However, there is no specification for those plans, no specification of who is responsible for following through, and no indication of who will pay for the care. Apparently no one monitors hospitals to see that such discharge plans are made, much less carried through (Comptroller General of the U.S., 1977).

Medicare was a medical program, based on a medical model, with limited financing for psychiatric care for fear of its long duration and excessive costs. Financing for psychiatric care was not considered separately from financing of other medical care, and undoubtedly reflected the politics of Medicare-Medicaid legislation. Getting the legislation passed at all required great courting of medical interests who had long opposed anything resembling socialized medicine. In order to gain the support of organized medicine, reimbursement formulas were exceedingly generous (Stevens & Stevens, 1974). At the time, it would have been unthinkable to include other than medical model programs in the legislation. To this day, for example, care rendered by a licensed psychologist is still not independently reimbursable under Medicare. We are still living with the consequences of that decision, which might have been necessary as a compromise to gain the greater good of general medical coverage for the aged and the indigent.

Medicaid. Medicaid is a federally sponsored program to provide health and rehabilitation services to the needy, including the medically disabled. In contrast to Medicare, considered an insurance program, Medicaid is a welfare program, with all of the problems attached to welfare programs. The program reimburses states for allowable costs of services provided to eligible individuals. The federal government reimburses states at rates ranging from 50 percent to 78 percent. Medicaid legislation limits care in mental hospitals to those over 65 or under 21. All those between 21 and 65 who are eligible due to disability or to their state of indigency can receive inpatient psychiatric services in a general hospital. Each state defines the extent of benefits it will provide under Medicaid, so long as federal guidelines are met. In effect, there are 53 programs. Generalizations are hazardous.

Medicaid has helped to empty the state hospitals, especially of the elderly, although they still constitute some 30 percent of public mental hospital patients (Task Panel on Costs and Financing, 1978). Medicaid funds were used to move elderly mental patients from state hospitals, where the state paid the full cost, to cheaper nursing homes, where costs are shared with the federal government. Between restrictive admissions practices and wholesale discharges to nursing homes, it is now true that more mental patients reside in nursing homes than in public mental hospitals. (See below for a more detailed presentation of data on this point.)

Nursing homes and intermediate care facilities were used because the states could receive partial federal reimbursement for patients residing in them. The average monthly cost of maintaining patients in a mental hospital is around $1000 a month, and in some states as much as $2000 a month (U.S. Senate Subcommittee on Long Term Care, 1976). State hospital costs come out of the state's mental health budget and are financed exclusively with state revenues. A state can reduce its costs substantially by placing a mental patient in a nursing home or in an intermediate care facility whose total monthly charge might be a third of the costs of the mental hospital, and the state would be reimbursed at least 50 percent of that amount from the federal government. If the intermediate care facility cost $374 a month and the state received a 68 percent reimbursement rate, then the net cost to the state budget would be $120 a month, and it would be shifted from the mental hygiene to the welfare budget.

Presumably facilities receiving Medicaid patients are regulated. However as the U.S. Comptroller General (1977) and the

U.S. Senate Subcommittee on Long Term Care (1976) pointed out, in most places there is no regulation worthy of mention, and abuses abound. In addition, the Comptroller General (1977) believes many placements were made in violation of legislative and HEW regulations. We shall return to the problems of abuse below. First it is necessary to review another government program that has contributed a financial incentive to the states to deinstitutionalize, the Supplemental Security Income Program, or SSI. In another section below, we shall show how these programs literally created a profit-making industry to care for individuals formerly cared for in state hospitals.

Supplemental Security Income (SSI) and community based care. While Congress sometimes provides programs and funds that are well intended, it often happens that the intentions are subverted as funds are used to meet some other bureaucratic objective in the course of implementing the legislation. The 1965 Social Security Act had several programs to provide services to families with dependent children, to the aged, the blind, and the disabled. Established for the purpose of helping needy persons attain or retain the capability for independent living, reimbursable services included payment for placement in foster homes and halfway houses among other things. The programs were important because they could finance placements for those not eligible for Medicaid or Medicare. However, the funds were used to support the elderly and the disabled in residences that could not meet federal standards for Medicare reimbursable facilities. They were used because better facilities were not available, and it was cheaper to maintain patients in those settings than hospitalize them. The U.S. Senate Subcommittee on Long Term Care described the way it worked:

> The key to the "dodge" is that the States maintained the fiction that the individuals in question were independent. Old age assistance checks, of course, were cash payments addressed to qualifying individual payees instead of "vendor payment" which would list the nursing home as payee. In fact, the individual would endorse his check over to the facility owner (often the endorsement was accomplished by the owner making an "X" on the back of the check). (p.724)

Because of the abuses which came to light, Congress in 1972 changed the law so that states could receive reimbursement for such efforts only through the Medicaid program (PL 92-603). By making payment directly to the vendor (the proprietor of the home), the facilities would have to meet the none-too-stringent standards set for Medicaid reimbursable services of this kind. What is incredible is that the Congress turned around and did exactly the same thing in another part of the same bill they had corrected in the first place. Seeking to consolidate assistance to the needy, to the disabled, and to the blind, and seeking to bring the states to some minimal and more nearly equitable level of assistance granted to each person in need, Congress passed the SSI program, wholly funded by the federal government. SSI provided a floor of $130 a month under the incomes of the blind, the disabled, and the aged poor who were ineligible for other social security pensions, or who received less than that. By 1976 the minimum had been raised to $167.80, and by 1980 it was still only $238.

If a state had been paying more than the minimum, and it desired to participate in the program, it had to guarantee that it would add sufficient amounts so that the recipient would not have less than he or she had before. However, if a state had been paying *less* than the federal minimum, any addition to the person's stipend was left to the state's option. It was theoretically possible for states now to divest themselves entirely of responsibility for contributing to the support of persons in those categories of need.

SSI had three features that contributed to the exodus of the elderly and those who could be classified as disabled from state institutions. First, SSI payments were barred to those residing in public institutions. Second, SSI payments were reduced by one-third if an individual lived with a relative. Third, SSI funds went to the individual as a direct cash grant. Since the older person receiving the benefit is theoretically a free agent and can choose to spend the money as he or she sees fit, welfare agencies were not obliged to exercise any control over those who provided services to the elderly or the disabled.

Just as Medicaid created a relatively unregulated nursing home industry (see below), so this amendment created a boarding home industry. To put it simply, the income allowed individuals to be released from institutions and to be placed in substandard boarding homes. The operators of some of these homes simply maximized their profits by crowding as many as they could get by with into substandard facilities, and then saving on the costs of food (Comptroller General of the U.S., 1977; U.S. Senate Subcommittee on Long Term Care, 1976).

With the passage of SSI, many states that were already paying less than the minimum in old-age and disability assistance ceased their contributions entirely. A few other states added some funds to bring the monthly stipend up to as high as $400. SSI payments could not be made to individuals in institutions, and there were other regulations favoring the course; states found it cheaper simply to discharge individuals outright from institutions. Such persons were often placed in unregulated board and care homes, or in single room occupancy hotels (SRO) with no obligation on the part of the proprietors to provide any service whatsoever.

While the rules are in the process of change, whatever the current situation, it is clear that states took advantage of the opportunity to remove patients from state supported facilities, (e.g., the state mental hospital) and place them in less expensive facilities, where the costs were carried in large part or entirely by the federal government. Patients were placed in unregulated facilities, where it would not be unfair to say that they were more or less sold to the lowest bidder. The U.S. Senate Subcommittee report and a New York State legislature report (Stein, 1976) provide ample evidence of the poor living conditions available for many ex-patients.

Before going on, a brief historical digression is in order to demonstrate that the nursing home industry itself had its origins in the 1935 Social Security Act meant to provide old-age assistance to those who had nothing.

The 1935 Social Security Act and the birth of the nursing home industry. The problems that emerged after the 1965 and the 1972 Amendments to the Social Security Act were replications of the problems that emerged after the passage of the Social Security Act in 1935.

The history of welfare begins with the break up of feudal estates at the end of the Middle Ages, a process of social change that made more visible a large underclass of the unemployed and the unemployable. Prior to that time, the aged, the disabled, the blind, widows, unwed mothers, orphans, illegitimate children, the insane, and the severely retarded were the responsibility of the manor, the community in service to the lord of the manor, and the local church. The Elizabethan Poor Laws of 1597–1601, laws which the colonists brought with them to America, were the beginnings of a formalized system of care for this underclass. Advocates of "indoor relief" (care in institutions) and "outdoor relief" vied with each other over the centuries, the popularity of the policies seesawing as each approach produced either its welfare scandal or politicians pointing with alarm to rising welfare costs.

Some form of institutional care was always necessary. In both England and in the United States almshouses and workhouses were major holding centers for the care of this underclass. In fact the French institution in which Pinel initiated the modern psychiatric era by removing the chains from the insane was just such a place of confinement. In nineteenth century America, the poorhouse was intended to be a miserable place, so that only those in direst need would avail themselves of the facilities. In order to avoid the degredations of the poorhouse, honest workingmen were supposed to be inspired to save to avoid entering its doors. "Reverence for God, hope of heaven, and fear of the poorhouse" the saying went. The proponents of the poorhouse succeeded admirably in one aim—people did fear the poorhouse. Since workers with marginal incomes could not save for their old ages, and private and public pensions were either nonexistent or thoroughly inadequate, horrible conditions did not prevent aged, sick, helpless people from entering those institutions, for they had no other recourse.

The Social Security Act of 1935 (PL 74-531, Sec. 3(a)) excluded poorhouse residents from receiving federal Old Age Assistance benefits. The intention was good—to eliminate the poor farms, known to be dread places providing scandalously poor care. The architects of the Social Security plan did not want to support the poorhouse. Within a surprisingly short time after passage of the Act, at least 16 states reported a notable reduction in the county poorhouse or poor farm census. Where did all the residents go? Many who qualified were placed on assistance and released into the community, or placed in boarding houses. The deinstitution-alization of the day correlated closely with reimbursement calcu-lations. If the state's per diem cost for maintaining an individual in an institution was more than the per diem cost of providing matching funds to place the person on assistance, then the person was placed on assistance and released into the community.

Three problems, very familiar to contemporary students of deinstitutionalization, emerged. First, severely ill persons could not be placed in the community; some county homes came to be infirmaries for the incurable. Second, when the county poor farm was entangled with local politics, and contracts for food, services, and other materials, and patronage-controlled staff positions were at stake, there was political opposition to closing the institution. Poor farms did not close. Many were still providing unconscion-able living situations for those unfortunate enough to be incar-cerated there as late as the 1950s. Third, substandard boarding homes sprung up. The boarding homes caring for the elderly often hired nurses, because the state would pay for such assis-tance to sick elderly, and eventually many of these grew into private, profit-making nursing homes. There was little enforce-ment of existing regulations and plenty of incentive for proprie-tors to increase profits by minimizing costs. There was little incentive for providing decent care, and few penalties for not doing so. Despite official knowledge of their inadequacies, few homes were closed down because welfare workers had no alter-natives. Closing down inadequate homes would literally mean putting sick people out on the streets. While few spoke up for the poor and the helpless, the operators of proprietary homes orga-nized and were able to influence public policy at state and national levels. When in the 1960s and afterwards the federal government acted to provide medical assistance for the elderly, the provisions of the various acts and reimbursement formulas were such as to encourage states to pay for extended care in private nursing homes. The 1935 Social Security Act had created conditions that were later to influence the deinstitutionalization process.

The conflict between humanitarian and economic values. The legislative history accompanying PL 92-603, the Act establishing a figure of $130 a month as a suitable payment under SSI, summarizes the House and Senate Committees' thinking about various provisions of the bill. There may have been testimony about what $130 a month would buy in 1972, but if there was it was not reported in the legislative history. Although the legislative history takes note that previous legislation was misused to support the "wholesale and indiscriminate transfer of patients from skilled nursing homes to intermediate care facilities" (p.5097), it is clear that the intent of the legislation was to *encourage* the transfer of patients to less expensive facilities (p.5059). There is not a word in the Act, and hardly a word in the legislative history, to express the Congressional intent that individuals live in dignity, in decent surroundings, and with adequate care. As an historical oddity, we might note that the phrase "a reasonable subsistence compatible with health and decency" was removed from the 1935 bill at the insistence of a southern Senator, who, in defense of state's rights and in fear of federal intervention in the treatment of blacks in the south, insisted that the phrase be replaced with the term "As far as practicable under the conditions in each state." It is a fine irony to think that the many white residents of inadequate nursing and boarding homes might owe some portion of their mistreatment to a decision based on racist considerations (Witte, 1962, pp.143-44; Altmeyer, 1966 p.39).

Since SSI was meant only to supplement other sources of income, the legislative history has an extensive discussion of the problem of determining how much other income a potential recipient might have. If a married couple lived together, and both were getting disability or Old Age Assistance payments, their income should be reduced, since it is cheaper for two people to live together. In its wisdom, the Congress determined that the value of room and board for people who lived in the home of a friend or relative was sufficient so that payment should be reduced by one-third. There was a discussion of whether the income value of a home vegetable garden should be counted in determining the actual benefit to be paid. We will not dwell on the politics of SSI which allowed those states already providing less than $130 a month to provide still less. The legislative history doesn't even express the pious hope that states would seek to do right by their needy elderly and disabled citizens. We should remember that the economists, the budget officials, and the social service experts are the modern descendants of the scientifically oriented Charity Organization Societies who intended to distinguish the worthy from the unworthy poor and to provide only what the worthy poor needed to survive (Levine & Levine, 1970).

The positivism of influential economists who view the economy not in terms of the lives of individuals, but in terms of mathematical models that generate the unreal figures of the Gross National Product (GNP), presents a real contemporary problem. Fuchs (1968), for example, discusses the problem of measuring productivity in health care. How does one measure the dollar value of changes in the level of health? By examining age adjusted mortality rates, one can reason to the dollar value of a decrease in mortality by examining the relationship between health and work output per man hour. One can add in the increase in productivity attributable to a reduction in the death rate, and a consequent increase in the labor supply. It is worth quoting Fuchs to understand the full implications of the economic view of the worth of a human being.

> The capitalized value of the increase, at a given point in time, can be obtained by summing the value of future potential earnings discounted at some appropriate rate of interest. The details of such calculations vary greatly from one investigator to another, but one result is common to all: the value of a man (in terms of discounted future earnings) is very different at different ages. It rises steadily from birth and reaches a peak at age 30 to 35. Peak values may vary from two to ten times the value at birth depending upon the rate at which future earnings are discounted. After the peak, *values decline steadily and approach zero at very old ages. The principal implication of the age-value profile is that the economic return of saving a life is not the same at all ages.* (emphasis added; pp.120–21)

If Congress was following economic advice based on such principles, it is clear that we need not concern ourselves with saving the lives of the elderly and the disabled, for they have no contribution to make to the economy by working. Of course they do make a contribution to our economy, increasingly based in the delivery of services as Fuchs' (1968) book demonstrates, by their necessary presence as the subjects of care delivered by others who are working by delivering the care. How would the boarding home and nursing home industries contribute to the GNP without the elderly and the disabled?

SUMMARY

While the community mental health centers program had its theoretical and conceptual origins in the writing and thinking of psychiatrists, psychologists, sociologists, and other professionals knowledgeable about the potentials for delivering care to people called mental patients, the program itself was shaped by the politics of medicine, by legislative compromise, and by the realities of the matrix of services and local governmental interests. The problem of caring for mental patients is part of the larger problem of welfare in a capitalistic and individualistic society, and funds to implement programs for assistance to the elderly and the handicapped depend upon welfare economics and health care economics and politics. Programs and policies that interacted with mental health programs and shaped them developed without any apparent consideration for the effect of one piece of legislation on another, and without regard for the tendencies of bureaucracies to pursue their own ends, almost independently of legislative intent or authorization. Everything is connected to everything else, ideas to politics, politics to economics, economics to bureaucratic organizational dynamics. One cannot understand one without looking at all the others.

Chapter 4

THE COMMUNITY MENTAL HEALTH CENTERS MOVEMENT
Achievements and Failures

There is little doubt that the community movement has achieved President Kennedy's goal of halving the institutional population. The population of our state hospitals has declined drastically, from about 559,000 in 1955 to about 160,000 by 1978. There has been a less drastic decline in the population of our institutions for the retarded. In 1968, the institutional population reached a peak of 193,200. It declined slightly to 181,000 by 1971, and since than has declined still more to about 155,000 in 1976 (Comptroller General of the United States, 1977). The decline in the institutional population tells only a part of the story. What happened to the patients? How did they fare in the community? In 1975 Congress found that the Community Mental Health Centers program was successful and worthy of continued support. How well grounded was that Congressional finding of fact?

The aged population of state mental hospitals. On any given day in 1969, there were 427,799 patients in state and county mental hospitals. Of these, 32 percent were over age 65. By 1974, the average daily census of mental hospitals was reduced to 237,692. In 1974, patients over 65 constituted 25 percent of the hospital population. While the state hospital population overall was reduced by 44 percent, the population over 65 declined by 56 percent; the population under 65 declined by 39 percent. The elderly patients went into nursing homes. Of all the elderly who were in some institution, the percentage in state mental hospitals declined from 30 percent to 12 percent in the decade from 1960 to 1970. The proportion of the institutionalized elderly who were in homes for the aged increased from 63 percent to 82 percent (Redick, 1974).

A very high proportion of the institutionalized elderly have some kind of mental disability. Estimates of the frequency of psychiatric disorder in the over-65 population range from 8 percent to 25 percent, depending on the definition of disorder. About 45 percent of those over 65 in nursing homes have a diagnosis of chronic brain syndrome, neurosis, or psychosis. One survey indicated there were nearly 900,000 residents in nursing homes with various mental disabilities including all degrees of senility. Another study estimated that 74 percent of the institutionalized elderly had mental disabilities of some consequence. Twenty-two percent of residents of nursing homes are under 65. Of these, 20 percent are mentally retarded and another 20 percent are mentally ill. Of the 900,000 residents with some degree of mental disability, 72,700 were under 65.

By any reckoning, there are now more mental patients in nursing homes than there are in state mental hospitals. (Comptroller General of the U.S., 1977). It is difficult to determine the number of patients in other publically supported facilities, intermediate care homes, halfway houses, boarding homes, and in private facilities, such as the single room occupancy (SRO) hotel, where the former patient's total support comes from government funds. Examined alone, the drop in the state hospital population is deceptive. Many former state hospital clients have simply moved over to other facilities where the financial burden has been shifted from the state's budget to the federal government's budget.

The elderly, the fastest growing segment of our population, generally have great need for care and assistance. The baby bulge of the fifties will become the senile bulge after the turn of the century. The figures are instructive. In 1950, those over 65 constituted 8.1 percent of the population. By 1980, there were over 24.5 million over 65, constituting approximately 11 percent of the population (U.S. Bureau of the Census, 1976, Table 3).

Many elderly have serious, disabling illnesses, and others are limited in care they can provide for themselves. As a consequence, and in the absence of adequate community supports, there has been an increasing demand for nursing homes, domiciliary and similar facilities. In 1964, there were 554,000 residents in such homes, but by 1974, there were nearly 1.1 million (U.S. Bureau of the Census, 1976, Table 133). Although the United States institutionalizes a larger proportion of its elderly than do other nations, it might be tolerable, or even desirable, if decent care was provided in smaller, community based facilities where the stigma of being a resident in a mental institution was reduced, and where residents could take advantage of community living to the degree they were able. We have never planned adequately for our elderly. Again, ironically, the architects of the Social Security Act believed that the elderly who were chronically ill could be cared for adequately in our state hospitals. Ten years later the state hospitals were called snake pits, and twenty years later we heard the cry to remove the elderly from state hospitals where they did not belong. Although facts in abundance are available, we have never, as a society, faced the problem realistically (Levine, 1979).

Provision of care for the elderly and the disabled was a growth industry, particularly after the passage of the Medicaid Act, which provided a stable source of income for private proprietors. Investment counselors urged investment in nursing home chains at the time the legislation was drawn (Butler, 1975; Moss & Halamandaris, 1977). From 1960 to 1970, the number of nursing home patients increased by 210 percent, employees by 405 percent, and expenditures by 465 percent. By 1976 expenditures reached 8.5 billion dollars. That the industry was profitable is shown by the organization of large corporations to provide care. In 1972, 106 publically held corporations provided 18 percent of all beds and accounted for 33 percent of the industry's revenue. From 1969 to 1972, total assets of these corporations grew 123 percent, gross revenue 150 percent, and average profits, 116 percent. Similar profits were shown by individual operators as well, and in some instances, legislative investigation revealed gross profiteering (U.S. Senate Subcommittee on Long Term Care, 1976).

Reimbursement rates are fixed by law in the Medicaid program, based on formula for determining costs, or in the case of those receiving SSI, by the amount of the stipend. Profit-making proprietors can increase profits by reducing costs. Costs are reduced by reducing the level of care to patients. In some cases, it seems we have come but a short distance from colonial times when mental patients were auctioned off to the lowest bidder (Deutsch, 1949).

Homes participating in the Medicare-Medicaid programs were supposed to be supervised by state departments of social service and state departments of health. Supposedly they met federal standards for personnel and physical facilities. However, there was no mechanism for federal enforcement and HEW regulations were characterized as "so vague as to defy enforcement." A few states did a good job, but in many enforcement was nonexistent, or scandalously ineffective. In addition to the 16,000 facilities participating in Medicare and Medicaid, there were 7200 non-participating facilities, subject only to whatever regulation local health or fire safety authorities might see fit to impose (U.S. Senate Subcommittee on Long Term Care, 1976).

In consequence, care is exceedingly poor in many facilities. Physicians are not often interested in geriatric problems. Fees for visits to nursing homes are relatively low, payment is bogged down in red tape, and current standards require only infrequent visits by physicians. Existing regulations do not specify any ratio of nurses to patients, and about a third of the facilities are not required to have a nursing officer on duty at all. In consequence there were only 65,235 Registered Nurses in 23,000 nursing homes (recall that 24-hour, 7-day-a-week coverage is necessary), and their turnover rate was 71 percent per year. Unlicensed, untrained, low-paid orderlies and aides provide 80 to 90 percent of the care, and the turnover for these persons is about 75 percent per year.

Many abuses follow. In 1973 there were 6400 nursing home fires. An estimated 500 patients lost their lives in those fires; 51 fires were severe enough to kill three or more people in the same incident. In 1975 an estimated two thirds of the 23,000 nursing homes had four or more deficiencies or violations of the Life Safety Code of the National Fire Protection Association. The U.S. Senate Subcommittee on Long Term Care reported that existing standards were not enforced in many communities.

Profiteering in unregulated homes results in crowding, poor physical facilities, low-paid help, and inadequate food. The U.S. Senate Subcommittee reported instances of patients living in chicken coops, and operators who set aside 54 cents a day per person for three meals. There has been cheating in addition to profiteering. Nursing home scandals periodically hit the front pages of newspapers with reports of operators who bill for non-existent services and medications. Pharmacists have been required to kick back to operators for the privilege of providing drugs. Thus welfare has been billed for nonexistent prescriptions, out-dated drugs, and drugs of questionable value. Generic drugs are supplied but the bills are for more expensive brand names. The mean annual bill for drugs was $300 per patient. Profitability is so good that a psychiatrist in charge of a deinstitutionalization pro-gram testified that he had been offered $100 a head to steer patients coming out of his institution into particular nursing and boarding homes (U.S. Senate Subcommittee on Long Term Care, 1976, p.726).

Almost 40 percent of drugs were painkillers, sedatives, or tranquilizers. Due to poor supervision and poor training, 20 to 40 percent of all nursing home drugs are administered in error, with a high instance of adverse reactions. Butler (1975) states the situation is compounded because we know very little about how elderly persons metabolize drugs. Nursing home patients are often tranquilized simply to keep them quiet and make it easier for the staff to care for them. Neglect and abuse has led to some deaths. Physicians do not routinely view the bodies of patients who have died before signing death certificates.

Investigators found residents fearful of reprisals if they com-plained of poor conditions. They observed verbal abuse and suspected physical abuse. In some settings, residents did cleaning and household and kitchen work with little or no pay and were thus exploited. Such unreimbursed services are not permitted of involuntarily committed patients in state hospitals. Patients required to work must receive minimum wages (*Souder* v *Bren-nan*, 1973). Many facilities showed no evidence of medical, psy-chiatric, or other therapies, or recreational programs. Patients were found sitting in their rooms, sometimes tied to their chairs. Theft of patient property and misappropriation of patient funds is commonplace.

Observers generally agree that patients were dumped, some-times by the busload, from state hospitals to nursing homes and to board and care homes. There was little screening and little fore-thought for the consequences. Goplerud (1979) reviewed the literature on the consequences of transferring the elderly to com-munity settings. Rather than promote recovery, deinstitutionali-zation of the elderly frequently triggered deterioration and even premature deaths, particularly of older, frail males who were cognitively disturbed. Elderly persons moving into less satisfying physical environments were also more likely to deteriorate. Gop-lerud points out that the available studies may underestimate the risks because most of the studies have been conducted in better than average facilities. Poor facilities don't usually open them-selves to study, and they are not usually affiliated with research organizations. Facilities such as the one studied by Henry (1963), aptly nicknamed "Hell's Vestibule" in which the proprietor remained one jump ahead of the Health Department, do not sponsor or cooperate with research on deinstitutionalization.

Nursing home industry problems are well described by Vladeck (1980), and those of board and care homes by the U.S. Senate Subcommittee on Long Term Care (1976). It is difficult to remain dispassionate when one reads the material, or visits such facilities. How much first-hand contact with the problems do legislators and government officials, who put together the pro-grams, actually have? True, they have professional assurances that geriatric patients do not need to be in hospitals, but the ones who make the decisions are state-level authorities who sit in huge commissioners' offices around polished board tables reviewing paper, and calculating how much could be saved. According to Goplerud's review, data were available by the early and mid-sixties showing that such moves could be dangerous. Yet it was only when scandals, fiscal and human, hit the headlines that legislators and bureaucrats moved at all. One wonders what such a person would feel, knowing that administrative actions designed to shift the burden of costs from one budget to another budget hastened the deaths of some of the persons involved.

Deinstitutionalization and funding for community services. While there are far fewer patients in state and county hospitals, and more patient contact takes place in outpatient settings in the community than in the hospital (68 percent of patient care episodes in 1973, compared to 23 percent in 1955) (U.S. Bureau of the Census, 1976, Table 86), community based facilities did not make much systematic contact with released patients. That was particularly true for the elderly. Those over 65 constituted less than four percent of admissions to CMHC's, and one center indicated it simply didn't accept patients over 60 for treatment (U.S. Senate Subcommittee on Long Term Care, 1976). Recent legislation (PL 94-637) contains provisions to encourage CMHCs to provide services specifically for the elderly.

Community mental health centers have provided little of the community based care to maintain patients in the community. Coordination between state mental hospitals and CMHCs, often established while bypassing state mental health authorities, has been inadequate (Legislative History, PL 94-637). Schulberg and Baker (1975) demonstrated that CMHCs have complex but generally distant relationships with each other. Since most funding for direct mental health services comes from state mental health departments, until recently, state supported community based care was rare.

The theory behind the Kennedy legislation was that resources would follow the patients, in the sense that its designers expected state mental health authorities to release funds along with patients to provide community based services. Instead, some states simply discharged patients to local communities in the hopes that necessity would become the mother of invention and local resources would be found. Patients would receive "administrative discharges." As might be expected, this strategy met with indifferent success. California, through its Lanterman, Petrie, Short Act of 1968 provided financial incentives to local communities to provide care. Even though local communities could receive nine dollars in state assistance for every dollar put into mental health facilities, local services developed slowly, and they were not always what chronic patients needed. The arrangements put local authorities into complex, and not always welcomed partnerships with state and federal authorities, relationships still being worked out (Robbins & Robbins, 1974; Lamb & Edelson, 1976; Aviram & Siegel, 1977; Levine, 1980). In New York, the state hospital system still absorbs the lion's share of the mental health budget. In 1976, $106 million was recommended for local community services, while $924 million was designated for "Regular State Purposes."

The decline in the state hospital population has not been accompanied by a decline in the budgetary allocation for institutional care. Nationally, expenditures for psychiatric hospitals have more than doubled those for 1965, even though hospital censuses have dropped by more than 50 percent in the same period (U.S. Bureau of the Census, 1976, Table 127). Large facilities have high overheads, and a reduced census does not reduce overhead by an equivalent amount. In addition, hospital admissions have increased so that even though the daily census has declined and patients stay in hospitals for shorter periods, hospitals are still very busy (Witkin, 1979).

In California, counties were charged for each patient sent to a state mental hospital. However, if a patient was released for community care, the local community received only half as much for after-care services, partly because of the problem of institutional overhead (Lamb & Edelson, 1976). One state hospital oriented toward community care decreased its census from 1826 inpatients to 590 inpatients; although in the overall it had fewer staff (1207 as compared with 1626), 85 percent of staff were still assigned to inpatient services (Levine, 1980).

Funding problems in developing community based care remain acute. The original CMHC plans called for a declining proportion of federal funds and an increasing proportion of local support. Local funds were to come from local and state taxes, patient fees, and third-party payments, including Medicare, Medicaid, and private insurance. By 1970, it was apparent that some local communities were jettisoning CMHC programs as their share of the costs increased. Congress found it necessary to extend the staffing grant program. Bass (1973) reported that older centers, experiencing a greater decline in federal staffing funds, derived a larger percentage of their funds from receipts from services. The 1975 CMHC Act Amendments provided additional funds for centers whose federal grants ended, but the dollar allocations have been insufficient, and the federal rescue funds were time-limited. Centers were urged in the 1975 legislation to become even more dependent upon insurers. However, insurers will cover inpatient costs and generally do not provide reimbursement for alternative community based services such as halfway houses and day care centers. Although practices vary state by state, inpatient care by physicians is covered and long-term care delivered by paraprofessionals is not. Where the innovative CMHCs were supposed to deliver innovative services, paradoxically, one set of government policies is being undercut by another set working at cross purposes with it. Landsberg and Hammer made the following prediction:

> To meet fiscal pressures, community mental health centers will increasingly emphasize inpatient services. Programs such as day hospital, day care or halfway house, and sheltered living will be deemphasized. Consultation and education programs, including prevention activities, will lessen in their importance despite special grants. Incentives for new and experimental types of clinical outreach programs will be nonexistent. The pressures to hospitalize and to rehospitalize patients will mount. Community mental health centers will, to a large degree become "revolving doors." They will become duplicates of the much criticized state hospital systems they were designed to replace, the only difference being that they are community based. (1977, pp.66–67)

The state hospital as a vested interest. While some state hospitals have shown vigor in reorienting themselves to new demands (Schulberg & Baker, 1975; Levine, 1980), changes are still slow. As a general rule, change has taken place primarily in a few urban centers affiliated with teaching institutions. Staffing patterns in state hospitals emphasize custodial care. In 1970, more than 80 percent of the personnel in hospitals were aides, attendants, clerical, fiscal, and maintenance workers. The technology of care is custodial, and in most places the staff are comfortable with the status quo and believe that changes would lead to increased problems without providing very much benefit to the patients. Demands for change tend to come from on high, from state-level officials, while those on the line, with de facto power, are less interested in and less involved in change.

Many in state hospitals see the changes as threatening to their employment and resist, actively or passively, on that account. Many rural communities are economically dependent upon the state facility as the major employer in the area. Shutting down a hospital could create a small economic disaster in some places, leading to political reluctance to close facilities. Given that many state hospitals are located in rural communities, it is necessary to take into account career people working in the system. Relocation programs, early retirement, and retraining have all been proposed and tried (Schulberg, Becker, & McGrath, 1976; Levine, 1980).

Expensive ads were placed in newspapers like *The New York Times* by the American Federation of State, County and Municipal Employees (AFSCME) to emphasize the worker's plight. Perlman (1976), an AFSCME official, points out that the union represents 150,000 mental health and mental retardation workers who not only have financial stakes in the mental health care system, but who are also concerned about maintaining good working conditions to enable employees to render decent service. However that may be, in New York State, union opposition to the state's deinstitutionalization effort ceased with an agreement between the governor and the union that 50 percent of the positions in the community as case managers and in outpatient facilities would be filled by state hospital employees.

Goldman (1977) presents some intriguing ideas about both the conflict and the mutuality of interests between mental patients and institutional employees. An institutional client requires approximately two caretakers, each of whom receives a salary and other benefits. If resources are shifted away from the institution toward welfare payments to maintain clients outside of institutions, employees may suffer. However, if the shift in resources is designed only to save money, and adequate services to support a decent life in the community are not provided, then patients and their families will suffer as well as employees. Goldman suggests a political coalition between patients, their relatives, and institution employees to seek adequate funding for varied services. Second only to patients, who are the recipients of care, line employees are most aware of the consequences of poor working conditions for patient care. Goldman maintains that the common enemy is the scarcity of resources, and suggests that patients, their relatives, and institutional employees band together to fight scarcity.

Community resistance. The wholesale placement of patients has created "psychiatric ghettos" in many communities, calling forth community resistance and well justified indignation. It is not only middle-class, well organized neighborhoods that have protested and attempted to block the location of community based facilities. A hospital in Massachusetts located living quarters for white patients in a black neighborhood. While the landlords were happy to receive the rents, other groups seeking to organize the neighborhood to deal with its myriad problems argued that the presence of chronic patients looking peculiar, dressing peculiarly, and sometimes hallucinating on the streets, added to the problems of the neighborhood (Schulberg, Becker, & McGrath, 1976).

In deference to the power of an organized neighborhood to protest, such facilities tend to be located in more transient neighborhoods with high rates of renters, high rates of moving, and low rates of home ownership. Fairweather et al. (1969) selected just such a neighborhood for their first lodge. The plan works out well, provided a particular neighborhood doesn't become saturated with large numbers of chronic clients.

Deinstitutionalization and the provision of community based services is a trend in other human service fields as well. Corrections, youth services, addiction services, alcoholism services, mental retardation agencies, and agencies for the aged are all interested in developing community based facilities. All look for the same type of marginal, transitional, or high-transient neighborhoods. Since each agency functions independently of the others, certain neighborhoods become saturated with social welfare clients. In Chicago, 13,000 ex-mental patients were relocated in an area called Uptown. In Washington, D.C., hundreds of patients can be found in the vicinity of Ontario Road, N.W. In Long Beach, New York, 3000 welfare clients and between 300 and 800 former mental patients were housed in the city's old hotels. It is estimated that 4 percent of the population in one area of the Upper West Side of Manhattan are recently released mental patients. Kirk and Therrien (1975) report similar phenomena in Hawaii.

In Buffalo, N.Y., the councilman for one city district received so many complaints about mental patients and others classified as having social problems that he sponsored a study of the area.

Two city neighborhoods housed 548 clients and former patients. While these constituted 54 percent of all clients in residences in the city, the two districts accounted for only 16 percent of the Buffalo population. The remainder of Erie county (the geographic district covered by the Erie County Department of Mental Health, the agency responsible for local mental health services), with one and a half times the population of the City of Buffalo, had only 42 percent of client residents in various care facilities.

The following agencies maintained residences in Erie County or in Buffalo:

New York State Department of Correctional Services (2 sites)
New York State Department of Mental Hygiene (146 sites)
New York State Division for Youth (8 sites)

Erie County Department of Mental Health Contract Agencies
   a. Transitional Living Services (17 sites)
   b. People Services to the Retarded Adult, Inc. (4 sites)
   c. United Cerebral Palsy Association of Western NY
Erie County Family Court
Baker Hall (residences for adolescent youth—3 sites)
Buffalo Boys Town
BUILD Halfway house (corrections)
Child and Family Services (2 sites)
City Mission (alcoholics)
Compass House (runaways)
Ingleside Home for Girls (emotionally disturbed and/or unwed pregnant adolescents)
Protestant Home for Children (4 sites)
Shiloh House (youth religious revival center)
YWCA (housing 85 former mental patients)

The two saturated neighborhoods had residences sponsored by 11 independent agencies. One agency, located in a neighborhood with four community residences, decided to open a fifth nearby. The agency touched all official local bases, and received approval for the additional residence. Six months later, yet another agency opened a facility four doors away from the newest residence without checking with any neighborhood organization, political representative, or any other agency officials. Neighborhood reaction was swift and negative.

No data are available on the large number of patients discharged, placed on SSI, and located in privately run boarding and apartment houses. No one monitors these patients since they are presumed to be independent. However, a great many locate in the vicinity of the Buffalo Psychiatric Center, the state hospital from which they were discharged. So many obviously psychotic former patients were wandering the streets that some businessmen in the main thoroughfare alongside the hospital, which is located in a city neighborhood, posted signs illegally barring patients from their premises. Administrators from the Psychiatric Center and the County Department of Mental Health and area businessmen had a heated meeting that resulted in a moratorium on further expansion of community residences within the neighborhood (Hoyt & Hopkins, 1976).

Even though it is difficult to organize a relatively disorganized neighborhood, merchants associations, block clubs, and other citizens groups eventually do complain to politicians, or their complaints lead to publicity and a public demand for action. In Buffalo, a coordinating council was developed following the meeting with the citizens' groups. The several agencies voluntarily agreed to minimize placement of their clients in the one district. In Long Beach, N.Y., public pressure and newspaper publicity resulted in an ordinance, of questionable constitutionality, banning the placement of discharged mental patients in the city's old hotels (U.S. Senate Subcommittee on Long Term Care, 1976). Such community resistance may well lead to a rethinking of deinstitutionalization policies.

The fear that mental patients will commit crimes is a factor in community feelings about releasing patients to the community (Miller, 1976). Some patients do become involved criminally. A person who urinates in the street may be charged with exposing himself. Another actively hallucinating, or shouting and gesticulating may be arrested for disturbing the peace. There is some evidence that the release of patients into the community has increased the rates at which former mental patients are arrested (Abramson, 1972; Zitrin et al., 1976). As communities become aware of the problems, there is increased pressure to accept patients into more protected settings. According to the Deputy Commissioner of Mental Health for Erie County, the number of persons charged with disorderly conduct and later committed to state hospitals tripled between 1975 and 1976 in Erie County (*Buffalo Evening News*, August 3, 1977).

The receptivity of a community to patients, and experience with them, can make a difference. A tolerant community, used to "characters" in the neighborhood, may watch with mild amusement as a former patient dances in the streets and disrupts traffic. Citizens of Geel, Belgium, with 700 years of experience in providing community based foster care for mental patients have very effective informal means of exerting social control to limit problems created by occasional odd behavior in public (Roosens, 1979). Scheff (1966) lists community tolerance as one of the variables determining whether or not odd behavior ("residual rule breaking" in his terms) is subject to social control and public labelling. So far, community mental health workers have engaged in a few, small experiments in attempting to win community support for their clients. It is a remaining task for community organizers to learn how to harness citizen sympathy and support to maintain patients in community residences.

Efforts to integrate services. Two important government reports, that of the Comptroller General of the U.S. (1977) and the U.S. Senate Subcommittee on Long Term Care (1976), as well as criticisms in the newspapers (e.g., Witten, Kerr & Turque, 1977; Koenig, 1978) have led to some rethinking of policy at the federal level. Fragmentation of responsibility, lack of clarity, and failure to define coherent policy is as pronounced in the federal government as in any other level, and perhaps more so because of its size. At present, 11 major federal departments and agencies are responsible for 135 programs that could provide service to the mentally disabled. The agencies control funds for direct clinical care, education, rehabilitation, employment, housing, and income support. There are federal programs to cover just about any need a mentally disabled individual might have. However, the agencies do not coordinate, do not cooperate, and tend to pursue their own priorities for program development (Comptroller General of the U.S., 1977). Despite a presidential message, and despite Congress' continued funding of the CMHC program, there is no formal, articulated policy labelled "deinstitutionalization" at the federal level. No single agency has the power or authority to coordinate policies and programs cutting across agency and cabinet lines. The coordinating mechanisms within the Executive branch fail to fulfill that purpose. Neither the managerial procedures used by the Office of Management and Budget (OMB); nor regional councils established in 1972 to promote closer working relationships between federal grant givers and state and local governments; nor the Under Secretaries Group for Regional operations, including representation from the Departments of Labor, HEW, Housing and Urban Development, Transportation and Agriculture, have succeeded in addressing the problem of interagency cooperation in deinstitutionalization. Mental retardation has fared only slightly better than mental health in getting some coordination within HEW, but agencies outside of HEW, and even many HEW departments do not cooperate in taking coordinated action. Two agencies within HEW, NIMH and the Developmental Disabilities Office, have responsibility for deinstitutionalization. They have no authority or influence over other HEW departments, much less over agencies responsible to different Cabinet officers.

Bureaucracies follow their own priorities and objectives. An NIMH official described the process of cooperating with another group to implement Title XX of the Social Security Act:

> While we were reviewing and commenting on issue papers we found out there were already draft regulations. When we were reviewing and commenting on draft regulations, we found out that regulations had already been published in the Federal Register. (Comptroller General of the U.S., 1977, p.46)

The lack of clear policy at a federal level complemented fragmentation at the local and state levels and compounded the problem of implementing Kennedy's bold new approach. The design to empty our large institutions was in part a response to a belief that large numbers of people were in them who didn't need to be there, and it reflected the view that large institutions were invariably bad (e.g., Goffman, 1961; Joint Commission, 1961). Labeling theory (Scheff, 1966) posits that the institution itself is partly responsible for the manifestations of chronic mental illness. However, deinstitutionalization was never meant to provide a rationale for discharging patients into the community, without further support, simply to save money. It meant, and means, changing the care of those who would be otherwise institutionalized from more to less structured living arrangements, from more dependent to less dependent living. It meant, and means, the development of satisfying alternative living arrangements and supporting services (Bachrach, 1976).

Comprehensive coordinated services are difficult enough to provide within a single institutional setting. Even in a hospital ward, personnel and therapists often are at odds about scheduling, for example. If disabled persons are to be maintained in a community, suitable living arrangements are required, and income support, training, employment, medical care, emotional support, and educational and recreational programs, as well as transportation, are all necessary. Such services are provided through separate agencies, each with its own administration, eligibility requirements, funding sources, and methods of providing the services. It is one thing to believe that large institutions are harmful, expensive, and unnecessary. It is quite another to promote a romantic ideal that fails to recognize the historical fact that the problems associated with dependency—poverty, aging, chronic mental illness, and mental retardation—have been with us since our earliest days. And it is still another matter to ignore the characteristics of government and of the social and political context in planning programs of care. It is not only that big government lacks coordinated policies and practices. Social scientists and mental health workers do not yet know how to think about the problems of planning and the problem of how the context affects whatever happens or doesn't happen. If this survey has demonstrated anything, it is how little we know or can anticipate the key variables that will influence our plans to serve. That problems emerged is less surprising than the fact that anything at all is accomplished.

In response to the Comptroller General's report and the U.S.

Senate Subcommittee's report, NIMH has attempted to cope with the problems. It sponsored a conference on community living for the mentally disabled in September 1976, and by January 1977 it had developed a draft of a proposal for a Community Support Program (Turner, Stone, & TenHoor, 1977). The previous strategy of training hospital staffs to take on new functions was seen to be inadequate, and the new strategy was to develop community support programs in the community. The chances for success in promoting some coordination in the community may have been enhanced by legislation (PL 94-63), which expressed congressional intent that CMHCs coordinate with other agencies. Although the legislation looks to the CMHCs to provide leadership in joint planning, service cooperation, and case management, CMHC directors have no authority to compel cooperation. In the absence of authority, there is no reason to believe that anything different will happen than has happened in the past.

The draft document for a Community Support Program was quickly translated into a small demonstration program. The agency responded to an immediate pressure with a program designed to show the agency was sensitive to Congressional wishes. Since then, the President's Commission on Mental Health (1978) has published its report, and an HEW Task Force reviewed its recommendations (HEW Task Force, 1979). The basic lines of community support are reflected in the Community Mental Health Systems Act recently passed by Congress. It is clear that government officials are now well aware of the criticisms described throughout this book. What is curious is that responsible officials didn't act earlier, on their own initiative. It took external criticism, and evidence of scandalous care, for bureaucratic officials to be able to act. Were they not aware of the problems before? If not, why not? If they were aware of problems, why do the reports made to Congress requesting additional programs read so positively? Why weren't the problems noted then? Was it a failure of research? Many of the problems of deinstitutionalization were first uncovered by newspaper reporters, and not by evaluation researchers. Are we supporting the wrong kinds of research? Is the political process such that it is responsive only to success stories or to scandal, but not to reasoned approaches to problem solving?

So far, there is nothing in either the President's Commission Report or the new legislation to show any fundamental approach to the problems of fragmentation. In the absence of a fundamental change, the most confident prediction one can make is that all the same problems will recur. Schulberg and Baker (1975) suggest there is some movement toward a unified human services agency concept in the field. Some (Chu & Trotter, 1974) have suggested that there be national social service insurance to replace all human service agencies. Bloom (1977) believes that the social policy underlying the CMHC Act and its several amendments may eventually evolve as a single, comprehensive, integrated community based health care system. So far the varied sources of funding for services and the separate agencies, each founded by separate legislation and each having different traditions and competing interests, have provided formidable obstacles to cooperation, much less to coordination and unification.

Given the difficulties of undoing history, it may be that we would be best off by accepting that our system is fragmented, and then do something not about the fragmentation, but about understanding how most of us make our way in this highly specialized society in which we are all dependent. As a middle-class, educated person with a modestly good income, and the willingness to be aggressive, I can usually cope without too much difficulty with most problems in living. Because I have knowledge, funds, and some social standing, I can find what I need, and when I find it, I am usually an acceptable client to the service deliverer. It may be that instead of trying to integrate services, we should do something about putting resources into the hands of consumers, and making available to them advisors who can help the consumers find and negotiate the necessities of life. I am thinking of something like case management and patient advocates, but with a consumer who has the resources to purchase services. As a popular advertiser says, "An educated consumer is our best customer." Perhaps we need to produce educated consumers of services who have the wherewithall to buy them, and in the absence of an educated consumer a consumer representative who can help the consumer make the free enterprise system work in the service arena. If we can't lick the system, we might find some way of taking advantage of it.

Lest our trek through the bureaucratic jungles prove too disheartening, let us now turn to an examination of some of the real accomplishments of the community mental health movement.

CARE IN THE COMMUNITY IS POSSIBLE

Despite the cynical and discouraging view one might develop about deinstitutionalization and community based treatment programs when viewed from a political perspective, it should not be forgotten that our large mental hospitals were, for the most part, rather terrible places. Alternatives in care needed to be developed to avoid for the future the major problems of inhumane care so prevalent in large institutions. There is good reason to believe that community based care is a viable alternative for many patients.

The theory of community based care is now fairly well worked out (Schulberg & Baker, 1970; Polak & Jones, 1973; Test & Stein, 1976; Kirby, Polak & Deever, 1977; Lamb, 1977; Anthony, 1979). Experienced practitioners believe they understand what is needed to provide the necessary services. In Lamb's words, "there is a considerable body of knowledge and techniques for effecting rehabilitation in community settings. What is needed is the will, the resources and the funding to do it" (Lamb, 1977, p.7).

A large number of studies confirm that the availability of community based services reduces hospital admissions (Emde, 1967; LaFave, Stewart, & Grunberg, 1968; Purvis & Miskimins, 1970; Sindberg, 1970; Weinman et al., 1970; Wolkon, Karmen, & Tanaka, 1971; Decker & Shealy, 1973; Doidge & Rodgers, 1976; Dawkins & Dawkins, 1978; Delaney, Seidman, & Willis, 1978). Literature reviews, covering these and many more studies (Anthony et al., 1972; Marx, Test, & Stein, 1973; Gottesfeld, 1976; Perry, 1978) generally conclude that community based services reduce the need for hospitalization, or reduce the recidivism rate by about half.

One study provided a natural quasi-experiment for the proposition that after care reduces the need for rehospitalization. Pasamanick, Scarpitti, and Dinitz (1967) demonstrated that a regime of drugs and support provided by community health nurses kept many patients from recidivating. Five years later, funding for the project was discontinued. A follow-up study showed that the original gains (three quarters of the experimentally treated group maintained at home) were eroded with the loss of the service (Davis, Dinitz, & Pasamanick, 1972).

Many of the components of a comprehensive system of care have been subject to evaluation. Thus Riessman, Rabkin, and Struening (1977) showed short hospitalizations were no less effective than long hospitalizations when judged by duration of patient stay in the community. However, many problems with the adequacy of the research limit confidence in that conclusion. Vannicelli, Washburn, and Scheff (1978) demonstrated that partial hospitalization programs were superior to full hospital programs, but neither diagnoses nor patient demographic characteristics predicted which patients would do well. Moscowitz (1980) recently reviewed the literature on day hospitalization and concluded that it is superior to in-hospital care. There is some evidence that it may reduce the likelihood of hospitalization postdischarge.

The increase in the number of community based facilities has resulted in a shift in the number of episodes of patient care from inpatient to outpatient settings. (A patient care episode is the entire treatment program for a single individual [Windle, Bass, & Taube, 1974].) There are problems in judging the significance of the shift. Community based programs may cater to select patients who are less difficult to treat (Michaux et al., 1973). Moreover, not all patients who are released make contact with aftercare services. The rehospitalization rate is lower among those who do contact aftercare programs, but the patients who are seen are a self-selected sample and might have done well anyway (McNees et al., 1977). Byers, Cohen, and Harshbarger (1978) arrived at a somewhat similar conclusion. On the other hand, Radinsky (1976) has demonstrated that within a comprehensive service, some 72 percent of transfers are successfully completed, showing that continuity of care is quite possible, when it is planned.

There is a substantial literature on alternative living arrangements (e.g., Colten, 1978) describing their uses for patients with differing needs. About 80 percent of patients adapt adequately in halfway houses (Rog & Rausch, 1975). They may provide important support for mental patients living in the community even after they leave the halfway house. Berman and Hoppe (1976) report that over 50 percent of released residents locate within one mile of the halfway house, and continue to use its facilities for formal and informal support. The research on halfway houses is not without critics who raise questions about its methods and its results (Cometa, Morrison, & Ziskoven, 1979). These critics agree that some clients, in some halfway houses, improve to some extent. They believe that more precise questions need to be answered.

In recent years, researchers using an ecological model have been looking at how the patient and the environment fit together. Thus Carpenter and Bourestom (1976) note that certain characteristics of the living environment promote retention in the community and enhance patient life satisfactions, McClain et al. (1977) have demonstrated that institutional and community based living arrangements have different atmospheres that could have significance for understanding the person-situation interaction in the placement of patients in community settings. Lehmann, Mitchell, and Cohen (1978) found that length of stay in a facility depends on the patient-environment fit. Nevid, Capurso, and Morrison (1980) have also shown that patient adjustment to family care is related to the discrepancy in the patient's perception of the living environment and what it is really like. Willer, Scheerenberger, and Intagliata (1978) showed that retention rates for retardates living in the community is highest amongst those released to group settings rather than to their own families or to other settings. Their findings have significance for the position taken by Arnhoff (1975) that deinstitutionalization stresses patients' families.

The poorest living settings are thought to be proprietary homes run for profit, and the so-called SROs, single room occupancy hotels, which house many former mental patients. There are some case studies of consultation programs to such settings that suggest that patient care and the patient's quality of life can be improved, if the mental health agency makes the effort (Levitt, Brownlee, & Lewars, 1968; Cohen, Sichel, & Berger, 1977).

The quality of life for former mental patients released to the community is a major issue. The value issues are not well clarified (see Levine, 1979), but the available research suggests that a reasonable number of patients do fairly well, although many live rather limited and restricted lives (Lamb & Goertzel, 1971). LaFave, Stewart, and Grunberg (1968) reported that on follow up, patients were doing well in community care, and there was no undue strain in the community. Purvis and Miskimins (1970) found that community based care resulted in an increased rate of vocational success and an increase in patient satisfaction with their care and their lives. Denner (1974) also reported patient satisfaction with community based treatment with care provided by people indigenous to the neighborhoods in which patients lived. Kirby, Polak, and Deever (1977) found evidence of considerably greater personalization of the environment and greater attachment by patients to personnel in community based, compared to institution based, services.

Christenfeld and Haveliwala (1978) sent student nurses who had expressed distinct reservations about community based care to visit community residences. They reported that patients in family care and in Adult Homes and Boarding Homes, although living in surroundings with an institutional flavor, valued their greater freedom. The student nurses, interestingly, had a much more dismal view of the situation when former patients were living in their own homes. The nurses thought the pathogenicity of the home continued and they feared for the eventual outcome of the placement although there is no follow-up data to confirm their fears. Moreover, many patients had social networks consisting almost exclusively of ex-patients, leading to questions of the degree to which they were truly reintegrated into the community. In the overall, the advantages of post-hospital living arrangements seemed to outweigh those of in-hospital living, and those advantages could not be duplicated in the hospital.

A critical problem in providing community based services is finding the means of reallocating funds from hospital based to community based care (Schulberg & Baker, 1975; Lamb & Edelson, 1976). Even when court orders require the reallocation of resources, compliance is often slow and incomplete (Lottman, 1976). The problems of change within bureaucratically organized systems subject to political control are extremely complex. Fear of the unknown aside, change is difficult because of ensuing losses in status, money, or advantage, in the amount or type of work people perform, and in working relationships. Union agreements, civil service constraints, budgetary cycles and their inflexibilities, and community resistance to having mental patients in their midst all contribute to difficulties in reallocating resources. It is widely believed that change in bureaucratic, civil service institutions is all but impossible.

However, in one situation a creative administrator, Yousuf Haveliwala, took over the directorship of an old line, rural, custodial state mental hospital and transformed it into a modern psychiatric center replete with an elaborate set of community based services. Haveliwala's approach to planned institutional change is described in detail elsewhere (Levine, 1980); briefly, his approach to change was data based. He made considerable use of program evaluation methods within a management by objectives framework. Relying on creative competition among his executives, he held them accountable for producing agreed upon changes. He had clear goals and objectives to which he held unswervingly, in the face of resistance from some of his own employees and from competing service providers in the community. His actions were always open, consistent, and consonant with clear objectives. He used his authority as chief executive to reassign people to positions of responsibility depending less upon formal credentials and titles, and more upon demonstrated competence in carrying out tasks. To make it worthwhile for people to work out of title and to accept responsibilities weightier than those for which they were paid, the Director used a variety of nonmonetary incentives.

Haveliwala developed community based facilities before releasing patients to the community. He found ingenious ways of reassigning hospital personnel to start outpatient settings before discharging patients. He reduced his hospital's census rapidly, and without "dumping," because support facilities were prepared before the patients left the hospital. The Director, with the support of his business and administrative personnel, was ingenious in finding budgetary flexibility even within the state's apparently rigid system. He bent, but did not break, rules to achieve desired objectives. While his programs were not without controversy, there is little doubt that he managed to transform the hospital from a predominantly inpatient service to a predominantly outpatient service, while maintaining and even improving inpatient care, as reflected in continued accreditation by the Joint Commission on the Accreditation of Hospitals, and all of this with a declining budget. Follow-up studies done by the hospital's program evaluators, complemented by special studies (e.g., Christenfeld & Haveliwala, 1978), and by an independent review (Levine, 1980) indicate that patients were being served by the latest techniques. Not only did the institution change, but there is reason to believe that chronic patients were afforded a decent life in the community, and they stayed there with relatively low rates of rehospitalization.

The Community Mental Health movement has by no means been a complete success, and there have been unconscionable abuses. However, the theory and practice is sufficiently well worked out so that it could be argued that if the facilities were in place, as the original architects of community mental health had envisioned, patient care in the community might well have demonstrated its merits. The barriers to implementation reflect political, economic, organizational, and professional forces that often work at cross purposes because of a lack of coordination and direction. As the Comptroller General (1977) pointed out so well, the Federal government entered this field without a well-thought-through policy.

The fault is less in the conception than in the execution. The failure of execution derives from an insufficient awareness of the political and social context within which change takes place. President Kennedy's promise to halve the census of state hospitals was made without thinking through the problem of what to do with those who are chronically dependent, a problem that has devilled western society since the break up of the feudal estates in the Middle Ages (Levine, 1979).

SUMMARY

This section has emphasized the problems in obtaining and coordinating services through fragmented government agencies. My criticisms do not imply the lack of necessity for services, nor should they be taken to mean that I am overlooking what has been accomplished. My criticisms are meant to point up deep-seated, recurring problems that will not be solved by official denial or professional blindness to the context in which services are delivered. Life is indeed a soap opera, and while personal networks provide sufficient support for many people, many others struggle alone with serious problems in living. Many of the problems outweigh the capacity of individual or family resources and require public services. The variety of outpatient services stimulated directly and indirectly by the community movement offer something to many who would otherwise have nothing. Outpatient services do not stigmatize as much as hospitalization does, and that advantage for the preservation of human dignity should not be dismissed. That innovative and preventive services have not yet developed is a problem for the future.

The evolution of federal involvement in mental health, traditionally a state function in our federal system, reveals that our problems, their definition, and proposed solutions all take place within a complex context in which political, ideological, historical, social, economic and psychological factors are inextricably intertwined. Large events—wars, immigration, social change, legislation, litigation in the federal courts—all have their impact in generating human problems. Sometimes solutions to problems generate new problems. But the specific social problems which come to our attention, the form in which they come to our attention, and the solutions that are proposed are far from being data based or based in the science of the day. The human fallout of social change is often treated as a psychological problem, amenable to care on an individual level.

The political structure, which allocates resources to the solution of social problems, has its own dynamics and its own mode of operation. The solutions must be congruent with what is possible within the complex interweaving of policy at different levels of government, and with separation and specialization of function. The power, status, and traditions of the helping professions are factors as well. Service to those in need is mediated by agencies and professions, and these have their own vital concerns. History also leaves its mark on the present. It is folly to ignore those residues of our past efforts to deal with deep-seated social problems. Every new initiative will inevitably encounter the old. Past is prologue.

Our narrow disciplinary orientations are insufficient either as a basis for understanding or for action, if we retain any belief in the possibility of programmatic solutions to problems on a national level. Now it may well be that large-scale, planned solutions are invariably chimerical and self-defeating. Perhaps, in accordance with the anarchist insight (Sarason, 1976), we ought to eschew centralized governmental solutions in the future. Sarason seems to agree with Kropotkin (1899) that any large-scale governmental effort will inevitably fail in the sense that it will reduce the psychological sense of community (Sarason, 1974), and reduce the sense of responsibility primary groups feel for solving the problems of their own members.

Be that as it may, whatever the direction of future solutions, we should be aware that whatever is done will be done in a social and historical context, which will have its impact. We cannot ignore the dynamics of the social context and think only in narrow disciplinary terms. To recognize the wholistic character of the system of which we are a part is most difficult, for it demands that we take distance from our own limited cultural and role perspectives, and see ourselves as participating in an elaborate and dynamic system. As we look more closely at the theories and the values that have guided programs in the twenty years past, and as we try to understand where we might go in the next twenty years, we need to keep in mind that the next generation of ideas and programs will be subject to the same forces. Our limited ability to understand, much less to control that context, should not limit our vision, but it should certainly increase the humility with which we approach our tasks.

Community mental health is not devoted exclusively to the care of the chronically dependent, although that is a large part of its mission. The preventive thrust that was so important a part of President Kennedy's message and vision is just now coming into its own, as reflected in one of the major recommendations made by the President's Commission on Mental Health (1978). (See Chapter 7, this book, on the President's Commission and its report.) Before going on, it is necessary to examine the effects on mental health care of successful litigation undertaken in the past twenty years. The legal system, the public interest bar, and activist judges have had their impact on the mental health system, and promise to have continuing effects in the foreseeable future. It is to that arena that we now turn.

Chapter 5

COMMUNITY BASED
SERVICES AND LITIGATION

"Is this enforcing the laws?
Nay, verily, it is merely making a wicked farce of it."

Mrs. E. P. W. Packard
Modern Persecution of Married Women's Liabilities (1875)

Mental health litigation has been among the most potent of forces making for change over the last fifteen years. As of 1975, there were over 100 completed or pending court cases adjudicating the rights of the mentally disabled. As of March 1976, there were court orders in ten states requiring the provision of services in the least restrictive alternative. Similar cases were pending in other courts (Comptroller General of the United States, 1977). Federal, state, and U.S. Supreme Court decisions have required greater constraint on involuntary admission of patients to institutions, required better care and treatment, and they have delineated the civil rights of patients in institutions. Under the theory of a right to treatment in the least restrictive alternative, federal courts have ordered far-reaching, and expensive, changes in the institutional care of the retarded and the mentally disabled, requiring the provision of alternative community based facilities.

In theory, mental health professionals approach the task of improving services in light of what contemporary knowledge and theory says is the best care. The legal profession is concerned with the statutory, common law, and constitutional obligations and rights of the various parties, and with feasible and enforceable remedies. While mental health professionals have cooperated with lawyers in framing cases and remedies, not all have been pleased with the outcome. Some believe the law has encroached harmfully on areas of professional autonomy. Those sentiments go back to the earliest days of lunacy legislation. Others fear that the law's focus results in paper victories for lawyers, which in the end may prove detrimental to patient care. Litigation has unquestionably been a significant force influencing the movement toward community based care, and while the results of litigation have often had important effects, too often the effects have been incomplete and fleeting.

The importance of the legal system for mental health care can best be appreciated by noting that until relatively recently, 90 percent of all mental patients were committed to hospital care involuntarily (Meyer, 1972) and the bulk of all patient care episodes took place in mental hospitals. It is only in the last decade that both of those figures have changed. Involuntary commitment is a judicial responsibility fulfilled through procedures that differ from state to state (Kittrie, 1971). Three purposes are served by judicial oversight of the commitment process. First, by following a prescribed process limiting compulsion, the individual is presumably protected from arbitrary state action that would deprive the prospective patient of liberty and of a good name. Second, the public is presumably protected from those who are dangerous to others. Third, individuals who were dangerous to themselves, or who lacked insight for the help they needed, could be brought to help.[1]

Despite the treatment rhetoric, the vast bulk of publically supported mental health care was provided in a coercive context. Commitment laws gave hospital officials virtually unlimited authority over their changes. In most instances, patients were released only on the say so of hospital officials. Patients lost many civil rights upon commitment. Indeed in some states commitment was tantamount to being declared incompetent, which in practice meant the loss of many basic citizenship rights including the

---

1. This chapter does not deal with criminal commitment nor with the insanity defense. See Goldstein, 1967; Kittrie, 1971; and Morse, 1978, for a discussion of those issues.

ability to enter into legal relationships such as contracts or marriage (Ennis & Siegel, 1973).

On the mental health side, all was done in the name of patient care, while on the legal side, it was done in order to protect society (the police power of the state) or to fulfill the state's obligations as the ultimate parent (parens patriae). As we became aware of abuses, inequities, and other unintended, deleterious consequences, an attack was mounted on two professional fronts. Mental health professionals and social scientists provided the theories, or the ideology if you will, and alternative designs for care. Lawyers fashioned legal weapons that when successful were backed by the court's vast powers of enforcement. That mental health litigation supported the community mental health objective of deinstitutionalization is not accidental. NIMH had provided financial support for legal studies and for litigation since the early 1960s (Kopolow et al., 1975).

While court decisions are couched in legal reasoning, social science thinking has had its impact. First, Thomas Szasz's books have been highly influential. His *Myth of Mental Illness* (1961) called into question the model of mental disorder as medical illness. He argued that mental patients were labelled as such because they violated legal, ethical, and social norms, and not because they had demonstrable lesions or physiological pathology. His later works, *Law, Liberty and Psychiatry* (1963) and the *Manufacture of Madness* (1970), were ringing indictments of the coercive mental hospital system and psychiatry's role in it. Szasz's work was even cited by the U.S. Supreme Court in *O'Connor* v *Donaldson* (1975).

Second, labelling theorists (e.g., Lemert, 1951; Becker, 1963; Scheff, 1966) formalized the concept that deviance was in the eye of the beholder. They advanced powerful arguments, and some evidence, that the public labelling involved in commitment, conditions in hospitals, and post-hospital stigmatization imposed formal and informal social disabilities, and in combination produced the chronic mental patient. Rosenhan's (1973) well known study was stimulated in part by the views of labelling theorists. Rosenhan was cited by the *Bartley* v *Kremens* (1975) court in support of its conclusions that the hospitalization of children was potentially deleterious, and that in the absence of the protections

of due process, mental health professionals acting for the state could easily deprive individuals of their rights to liberty and to a good name unnecessarily. No matter the evidence for and agains labelling theory the social science literature is used in legal brief (Ennis et al., 1975; Wald & Friedman, 1976) and is cited in cou decisions.[2]

Third, abominable conditions existing in mental hospitals an in institutions for the retarded in the post–World War II peri continued to exist in many institutions into the 1970s (Blatt Kaplan, 1966; Blatt, 1970; *Wyatt* v *Stickney*, 1972; *NYARC Rockefeller*, 1973). While some of the worst of the institutio cess pools have probably been cleaned up, one would no overly surprised to read a headline story detailing an instituti scandal in tomorrow's newspaper. Goffman's now classic l *Asylums* (1961) brought home the systematic impact institu had upon their inmates and influenced the thinking of c intervening in total institutions to bring about appropriate ch (Note Case, 1975). Ken Kesey's popular novel *One Flew Ov Cuckoo's Nest* (1962) publicized the overtly benign but co evil Big Nurse, and gave plausibility to accusations that patients might well have been harmed irreparably by the in mental institutions.

The professed aim of reform is to right wrongs and to in the care and treatment of patients. It remains to be seen h these goals have been met. While there has undoubted some success and a flood of literature on the relationship I the legal and mental health fields, it is not yet clear how interests of patients, their families, and the community h served. As yet we have but a handful of experiments in v courts have used extensive powers to bring about chan few experiments confront us with the complexity of about social and institutional change, and with the which mental health care is embedded in our total government.

One cannot understand developments in commur health without understanding the role of litigation.

2. See Scheff, 1966; 1975; Gove, 1970; and Murphy, 1976, for the d validity of labelling theory.

background, and to remind us that our problems are not ne
shall review briefly the history of commitment procedures
their influence on mental health practice in the United States.

HISTORY

The necessity for commitment procedures was recognized with
the opening of the first mental institution in Williamsburg, Virginia, in 1773. During the last half of the eighteenth century and
the first half of the nineteenth, not much more than a physician's
signature on a piece of paper was required to have someone
incarcerated. Some said minimal commitment procedures were
designed to keep paupers from signing themselves in to enjoy
institutional comforts.[3] In discussing the arguments against voluntary commitment, the New York State Commission in Lunacy
(1896) said: "One difficulty which attests this subject is the case of
those who would be desired to be committed at public expense
(p.136)."

Stimulated by the reputed success of moral treatment, public
and private mental hospitals and institutions for the retarded
opened all over the country. In general, the laws required that the
violently insane or the furiously mad be hospitalized, but not
much by way of procedure was required. An order by two
justices of the peace sufficed in many jurisdictions.

Given the laxity of commitment procedures, it was inevitable
that some would complain they had been railroaded into institutions by others with nefarious purposes, and that they had been
treated harshly while incarcerated. Confining people for their
own good always had some connection with economics. The
indigent insane were often confined in workhouses where their
labor could benefit the state. In England, the King's altruistic act
in assuming the guardianship of the well-to-do insane or the
mentally deficient also gave him the benefit of the profits of their
estates under early property law. With the development of mercantile capitalism, the imprudent use of property was taken as a
sign of insanity. Actions by relatives to involuntarily hospitalize

---

See Braginsky, Braginsky, and Ring (1969) for a modern description of a
milar problem in contemporary hospitals.

their kin were not infrequently motivated by the desire to preserve or control property. In the years following the establishment of mental hospitals the press carried stories by and about individuals who claimed they had been hospitalized without cause at the behest of relatives after their property, or because they were persecuted for other reasons. Mrs. Elizabeth Packard said she sold 500 copies of the book detailing her ordeal in a mental hospital when, in 1866, she testified before a crowded gallery to the Connecticut legislature.

Mrs. Packard's crusade in the mid 1860s was successful in changing lax commitment laws in a number of states. In 1860, Mrs. Packard had been committed to an Illinois state hospital by her husband, in conformity with a statute allowing married women and infants to be hospitalized at the request of the woman's husband, or the infant's guardian, without even the minimal evidence of insanity required in other cases. It took her three years to regain freedom, a story she told vividly in the two-volume book (Packard [1875] 1973). The book is a valuable first-person account of life in a mental institution, worthy of comparison with Clifford Beers' account some forty years later, and Ken Donaldson's story written a hundred years later. Following an episode that would rival the best in any dime novel, she was granted a jury trial, and when found sane, launched a national crusade to prevent the false commitment of others. Her efforts resulted in the Illinois "Packard Law" in 1867, requiring a jury trial to determine lunacy before anyone could be committed to an asylum. Other states also passed similar legislation about this time.

The history of Packard laws governing commitment should give pause for thought to those who seek the protection of individual rights by trusting to stringent due process. The Illinois Packard law required a jury trial prior to commitment. It also required that all those already incarcerated have jury trials within 60 days. We have no record of the immediate institutional response to the Packard law, which continued in force from 1867 to 1893. Professional commentators were dismayed by the results. Dewey (1913) claimed that more sane persons were found insane by juries, as shown by institutional reports, than were ever wrongfully committed earlier, including a number of muckraking journalists.

The Packard procedure was based in the criminal law. An individual accused of being insane was arrested, brought before the court, sometimes in manacles, and if convicted was taken into custody by the sheriff. Rather than subject loved ones to the rigor of jury trials, friends and relatives hid patients away until their disorders had become chronic and untreatable. The "depraved and unnatural acts and speech of otherwise respectable men and women were presented in open court." Goshen (1967) quotes an 1871 commentator who said:

> A harsh ordeal is laid down in this most singular statute. It converts every unfortunate person into a defendant in a prosecution, in which the dearest friends of the party, are, in the necessities of the case, converted into apparent enemies . . . there to be adjudged by the ignorant hangers on of the courthouse . . . what should be decided . . . upon the certification of a medical man is made to depend upon the haphazard opinions and caprices of men ignorant of the subject before them. . . . (p.166)

An 1889 commentator said that attorneys were assigned perfunctorily. The whole matter was conducted in a hurried fashion with some pains taken to conceal or obscure the fact that a trial was going on, so that the alleged lunatic was sometimes unaware of having been declared insane, even though fully capable of understanding the proceedings (Caplan, 1969). It took several years for the 1893 revision to take effect because Chicago courts continued to hold between ten and forty routine jury trials of alleged lunatics who were held in pretrial detention until lunacy trial day (Dewey, 1913). None of the commentators say anything about the legal fees to court-assigned attorneys, but one can safely guess that in Chicago, in those days, some function was served by the trials in addition to that of guaranteeing patients' rights.

A forensic profession sprang up with the tightening of commitment laws. So many physicians were called away from their hospital duties to appear as expert witnesses that the Board of Managers of the Utica, New York, State Lunatic Asylum (1873) complained that subpoenas were interfering with clinical duties. They also noted many of the problems modern critics find troubling:

. . . this matter of the testimony of experts, especially in cases of alleged insanity, has gone to such an extravagance that it has really become of late years a profitable profession to be an expert witness, at the command of any party and ready for any party, for a sufficient and often exorbitant fee. . . . One expert, whether real or assumptive is set up against another; and finally it will result that, by competition, pretended expertness will prevail, by numbers against the real expertness of these few thoroughly qualified men whose judgment is the mature experience collected from years of daily study and practical observation. . . . Such a perversion of the law and testimony results in constantly calling away from their public duties those who have a repute of superior skill and experience, who are often made witnesses under circumstances that impair the due weight of their opinions, and are adverse to a fair expression of them. . . . (pp.9–12)

Medical authorities argued that the various charges that they had railroaded the noninsane were unfounded, and that the involvement of courts simply aggravated matters. The Board of Managers asserted:

. . . commitments, to state hospitals . . . of persons who are not insane when committed, or who are detained after recovery, having been insane when committed, or who are not at once discharged when discovered to be sane, are so uncommon that not a case can be fairly vouched; and the final judgment in cases of *habeas corpus* . . . almost invariably result in returning the subjects of the writ into the same custody, often with an aggravation temporary or permanent of their malady caused by . . . their forced appearance before the officer or the court requiring their presence. (p.15)

The New York State Commission in Lunacy expressed the same concerns in its first Annual Report (1896). Dewey (1913), reviewing the Illinois Packard law experience, said that judicial inquest following its passage did not result in the discovery of a single sane person held in Illinois institutions. The New York State Commission in Lunacy felt the result was due to the necessity for a conspiracy between four persons: two certifying physicians, a judge, and the medical officer of the asylum, all presumably disinterested in the outcome would have to agree to commit a sane person, and they wouldn't agree unnecessarily. Modern research (see below) suggests that "conspiracy" is not that difficult to achieve. The Lunacy Commission, although protective of the system, gave some clues the system was not all that law abiding:

> Since 1874, the law has expressly required that . . . a casebook shall be kept. . . . In only a few instances was there even a pretense of keeping a casebook and in none was there found what the commissioners would regard as a proper casebook. (p.52)

Caplan (1969) believes that public attacks on mental hospitals and law suits against hospital superintendents (see Ordronaux, 1878) led to the demand for explicit commitment procedures, preferably under the superintendent's control, in contrast to the superintendents' previous stand in favor of informal procedures. To defend against future suits, hospitals began keeping records, but not for the purpose of improving patient care. The superintendents closed ranks against the hostile public. Hospital doors were closed, not only to keep patients in, but also to keep the public, including the family, out. The superintendents rationalized the limitation on family visits as necessary to prevent relatives or guardians from withdrawing patients from treatment prematurely. Isaac Ray ([1838] 1962), a foremost psychiatrist of the day, was fully in support of such limitations on public contact.

The increasing isolation of the patient, whether due to a desire to conceal deteriorating standards of care or to protect patients against their families, led to further court battles and legislative inquiry during the 25 years following Mrs. Packard's crusade. The newer laws, modifying commitment procedures, in fact did little to protect patient rights. The earlier laws, which contained no penalties for failure to observe them, were often ignored. An Illinois state investigation commission found 148 patients admitted to Illinois institutions without proper legal evidence of insanity (Packard [1875] 1973). Caplan (1969), however, believes that reform legislation in some other states resulted in improved conditions of care.

Problems existing before the turn of the century will be found to exist again and again in the modern era. Legal reform sometimes takes place in form and not in substance, leading to empty rituals that mock due process. Sometimes the reforms result in an emphasis on record keeping, a form of "defensive medicine" rather than treatment. Successful litigation may lead to court orders that are honored only in the breach, and they are followed by further litigation. The history of reform through the legal system should alert us to the hard realities that changing an encrusted and entrenched system having functional utility in society is not to be undertaken lightly, nor can quick, lasting successes be expected.

THE MODERN EPISODE OF LEGAL REFORM

Commitment laws changed with the emergence of professional psychiatry. Particularly influential was the emergence of forensic psychiatry as a discipline, to which the law could turn for assistance with difficult, intractable problems. Isaac Ray's book on medical jurisprudence, the first systematic treatise on the relation of the law to mental derangement, went through five editions from its publication in 1838 until the author's death in 1881. His ideas affected the thinking of lawyers and judges, and were influential in formulating the legal standard for insanity as a criminal defense. His discussion of the problem of determining insanity for purposes of civil commitment was highly lucid and still interesting. As Morse (1978) points out, the courts have the problem of balancing the individual's right to liberty and the assumption that each person is responsible for his or her own behavior, with the intuition that it is not right to treat a mentally disordered person like everyone else, when indeed the person may not be responsible. The decision presents moral, social, political, and legal dilemmas. Because the problems are difficult, members of the legal profession welcomed the opportunity to turn to scientific experts for their solution. Lawyers regarded incomprehensible behavior as phenomena beyond the bounds of their professional competence. They readily deferred to mental health experts. Because the medical model provided the rationale that confinement was for therapeutic purposes, for the good of the individual, commitment laws were made easier. The more rigid procedural rules were relaxed. Legislators also deferred to expert opinion in formulating codes governing commitment for mental disorder (Kittrie, 1971; Morse, 1978).

Professional mental health experts sought two goals in reforming commitment laws. They wished to make commitment procedures simpler, ostensibly to avoid trauma to patients and their families, and to retain involuntary commitment because it provided greater control over the patient while in the institution. Hospital authorites said it interfered with treatment and with management of the institution if patients could come and go as they pleased. In general, legislators followed the experts' recommendations. In some states, commitments were permitted without a hearing, simply on the sworn petition of a relative, a friend, an official, or any interested citizen, accompanied by a physician's certificate that the person was in need of care for mental illness. Commitments were for an unspecified period. Release depended upon the hospital director's judgment that the patient could function in the community (Kittrie, 1971). It was in this context of the arbitrary exercise of power and the attack on the inadequacies of institutional care that Szasz (1961; 1963) wrote his influential works accusing psychiatrists of being agents of social control.

The Baxtrom case and the prediction of violence. Coinciding with the beginning of community mental health legislation was the ending of the legal romance with psychiatry. The beginning of the end was *Baxtrom* v *Herold* 383 U.S. 107 (1966). Baxtrom, a convicted criminal, was committed from prison to a mental hospital for the criminally insane, but without having been afforded the protections of then-existing procedures for civil commitment. Convicted of second-degree assault, Baxtrom had served a little more than two years of a two-and-one-half to three-year sentence when he was transferred to Dannemora State Hospital, an institution used for the confinement and care of prisoners who became mentally ill while serving their prison sentences. Although his minimum sentence had been served and he was eligible for release, he was committed to Dannemora on the grounds that he still needed care and treatment in an institution. Although no qualified person said that Baxtrom required the security of an institution for the dangerously criminally insane, he was retained in Dannemora.

It took five years for Baxtrom's case to reach the U.S. Supreme Court. It held that Baxtrom had been denied equal protection under the law because he had not been committed following New York State's civil procedure. All other individuals in New York were entitled to a jury trial to determine their sanity, and confinement to an institution for the dangerously mentally ill required judicial review. Baxtrom had not had the benefit of such judicial review. Baxtrom requested that he be sent to a state hospital if he was in need of treatment, or that he be released. The Supreme Court agreed with Baxtrom and ordered judicial review of his sanity, as well as of all others confined under similar circumstances.

Following the Baxtrom decision, 967 others who had been confined past the termination of their criminal sentences were transferred wholesale to hospitals operated by the Department of Mental Health, or were released. Given the rapidity with which so many were transferred to state hospitals, it would appear the civil procedure was not much of a barrier to their commitments.

Monahan (1976) reviewed eight follow-up studies of Baxtrom patients, and a study of a similar situation in Pennsylvania (*Dixon v Attorney General of the Commonwealth of Pennsylvania*, 1971), which resulted in the release of 438 patients. Very few of the supposedly dangerous mental patients were involved in assaults either inside the hospital, for those who were committed, or outside, for those who were released. Four years later, fewer than 3 percent of the Baxtrom patients were in a correctional facility or in an institution for the criminally insane. After four years, half the Baxtrom patients were still in mental hospitals, but another quarter had been released. In four years, only 14 percent of the Pennsylvania patients had committed an act injurious to another person. McGarry et al. (1973) reported much the same for a group of Massachusetts inmates released pursuant to the Baxtrom decision. Monahan (1977) cautions that the "predictions" of violence were tested only after the subjects had been hospitalized for years. Short-term predictions of violence may be more accurate. The definitive experiment remains to be done.

The Baxtrom case broke no new legal ground in relation to civil commitment. However, the follow-up studies raised serious questions about the ability of psychiatrists to predict dangerous behavior. If patients convicted of crimes and held in institutions for the dangerously criminally insane had low rates of violence, what could one say about the validity of predictions of violent behavior in the case of others who had not yet committed any overtly violent act?

An important criterion to justify commitment of mental patients to institutions is the judgment that the individual is likely to be dangerous to others. Dangerous acts cannot be predicted with any certainty. Such acts have a low base rate, that is they occur infrequently. Any index, other than one predicting perfectly, would miss some who would act out dangerously, and it would also identify a large number of false positives, people predicted to act out violently who would not (Meehl & Rosen, 1955). Psychiatrists, working in public settings, are likely to overpredict dangerousness. Reasoning that it does little harm to hold someone for treatment, and that it does great harm to others, including the psychiatrist who is responsible for releasing someone who does harm someone else, they feel it is safer to commit someone to a mental hospital, or to hold a person who seeks release (Scheff, 1966).

The problem of predicting violence is a vexing one because of what is at stake: an individual's liberty on the one hand, and the safety and security of others on the other hand. Excellent reviews of the problem and the issues may be found in Miller (1976), Monahan (1976; 1977) and in Stone (1975), Stone being somewhat less pessimistic about psychiatric prediction than the other reviewers. Ennis and Litwack (1974) summed up the opinion of those who have reviewed the research literature on prediction in their subtitle: "Flipping coins in the courtroom."

When an individual charged with a crime is faced with the loss of liberty, the crime must be proven "beyond a reasonable doubt." That standard of proof is designed to prevent punishment of an innocent person, even at the cost of allowing nine guilty persons to go free. In the case of commitment to a mental institution, the individual may not yet have committed an overt act. The individual is committed on the basis of a judgment that he or she is likely to commit such an act. Monahan and Wexler (1978) have pointed to the ambiguities in applying the standards of proof to commitment situations, which until recently (see *Addington* v *State of Texas*, 1979) were settled on the basis of the easiest standard "preponderance of the evidence." If valid predictions of future dangerous conduct cannot be made, then it is clear from the research literature that a great many people have been confined unjustly, or had their confinements prolonged unnecessarily.

Due process of law. The primary protection for the individual against arbitrary state action is the requirement that the state follow due process. The protections of due process, although defined flexibly for different circumstances, include: the right to notice, specification of charges, right to counsel, right to present rebuttal, right to confront witnesses, and right to cross examine them. The juvenile courts, an American invention of the turn of the century progressive era, was meant as a reform of the then-existing practices of treating children as adult criminals, trying them in criminal courts, and confining them in prison with adults. Because the court, under its *parens patriae* power, was not to punish but to act as a wise parent toward a wayward child, juvenile courts dispensed with formal procedures and most elements of due process. If a child was confined under court order, it was for treatment, not punishment (Kittrie, 1971). Some of the early courts took their missions seriously (Levine & Levine, 1970), but the problems that later emerged were there from the beginning (Platt, 1969). Kittrie (1971) has an excellent discussion of the contemporary problem.

A year after *Baxtrom*, the U.S. Supreme Court voided much of the informal procedure used in juvenile courts (*In re Gault*, 1967). Gerald Gault, a 15-year-old, was committed to an Arizona state industrial school until he reached adulthood (i.e., until he was 21), on a charge of having made lewd telephone calls to a woman. Had he been an adult, the maximum penalty would have been two months. The Supreme Court said that the intent to help children through the juvenile court rarely had that result; informal judicial process contributed nothing but the violation of the constitutional rights of juveniles. The Court held that due process had to be extended to juvenile hearings. Subsequently, *In re Winship* (1970), the Court held that when a juvenile's freedom was at stake, the charge had to be sustained at the same level of proof used in criminal proceedings, beyond a reasonable doubt. Informal judicial processes, intended to help, were coming under increasing judicial scrutiny.

In 1967, the Court also decided in *Specht* v *Patterson*, that confinement of adults, even if to help, required a full panoply of due process protections. Specht, convicted of a sexual offense, was sentenced not for the offense itself, but was given an indeterminate term as a dangerous person. The Court held that he was entitled to a further hearing on the additional claim that he was a dangerous person. (Kittrie, 1971, discusses the problems of enforced therapy for sexual offenses both from the legal and the therapeutic perspectives.) This series of decisions said clearly that any deprivation of liberty required due process, whether it be termed civil or criminal, and whether or not it was for purposes of treating the individual or protecting society.

Competency to stand trial. On a national basis, a relatively small proportion of mental hospital admissions—approximately 3.4 percent in 1972 (Stone, 1975)—comes from transfers from prisons, following determinations of not guilty by virtue of insanity, or through adjudication of competency to stand trial. Brooks (1974) asserts the ratio of commitment for incompetency to stand trial to commitment following a verdict of not guilty by virtue of insanity is of the order of at least one hundred to one. McGarry et al. (1973) bear out this judgment for Massachusetts commitments. However, the situation with respect to adjudication of competency to stand trial varies from state to state. In Massachusetts in 1970, 14.2 percent of all admissions to mental hospitals were for observation. They quote a forensic psychiatrist in Colorado who claimed that the issue of competency to stand trial had been raised but once in his 17 years of experience.

Whatever the rate, nowhere was the potential for abuse more clearly revealed than in the situation in which a defendant, charged with a crime, was held for examination of his or her competency to stand trial. An extension of the premise that an accused be present at a criminal trial, the law requires that an individual be able to understand the nature and objectives of the courtroom proceeding, to understand the consequences at stake, and most importantly, to cooperate with counsel in a defense. When competency is questioned, a judge must decide whether the individual can stand trial, or whether it should be delayed until treatment has restored the individual to a sufficient state of competency so that a trial may be held.

The question of competency may be raised by either prosecution or defense. Judges tend to honor such requests, ordering the accused confined for psychiatric examination. Prior to 1972, it was not an unusual practice for prosecutors to raise a question about competency when the initial case against the defendant was weak. If an individual was found incompetent, he or she could be committed for an indeterminate period until treatment restored competency. It was not unusual for a prosecutor to drop the criminal charge once the individual had been committed. Many individuals were confined, sometimes for life, but often for many years beyond the maximum sentence that could have been imposed had the individual been found guilty of the crime (Goldstein, 1967; Brooks, 1974).

The Supreme Court attempted to correct the abuse inherent in the competency proceeding in *Jackson* v *Indiana* (1972). At the age of 27, Theon Jackson, a mentally defective deaf mute, unable to read, write, or to communicate except through the most rudimentary sign language, was charged with two robberies, one of $4 and one of $5. Jackson pleaded not guilty. When the question of his competency to stand trial was raised, he was examined by two psychiatrists who testified that due to his handicaps, he was unable to understand the nature of the charges against him, and couldn't participate in his own defense. Both said Jackson was unlikely to learn to communicate sufficiently well to stand trial, and another expert testified that the state of Indiana had no facilities to teach minimal communication skills to someone as deficient as Jackson. The trial court found him incompetent, and committed him to the Department of Mental Health until it could certify Jackson was sane.

The Supreme Court concluded Indiana could not commit Jackson indefinitely because of his incompetency to stand trial. He could have been released more readily if committed as a feebleminded person, or if subject to civil commitment as a mentally ill person. The Court held Jackson was denied equal protection under the law because the pending criminal charge subjected him to a less stringent commitment procedure and a more stringent standard of release than applicable to others not charged with criminal offenses. He had been condemned to permanent institutionalization without the state showing he had to be committed. The Court took notice that many defendants committed before the trial were never tried, and that they had longer hospital stays on the average than those committed through ordinary civil procedure. The Court took a dim view of the care and treatment available in most institutions to aid a defendant in attaining competency.

The Court seemed to invite further challenges to the states' powers to commit persons found mentally ill:

> The States have traditionally exercised broad power to commit persons found to be mentally ill. The substantive limitations on the exercise of this power and the procedures for invoking it vary drastically among the States. The particular fashion in which the power is exercised—for instance, through various forms of civil commitment, defective delinquency laws, sexual psychopath laws, commitment of persons acquitted by reason of insanity— reflects different combinations of distinct bases for commitment sought to be vindicated. The bases that have been articulated include dangerousness to self, dangerousness to others, and the need for care or treatment or training. Considering the number of persons affected, it is perhaps remarkable that the substantive constitutional limitations on this power have not been more frequently litigated. (*Jackson* v *Indiana*, 1972, pp.736–737)

Stone (1975) believes the Supreme Court's surprise was somewhat disingenuous. In previous years, the Court repeatedly refused to review cases challenging either the manner of commitment or of release. However, the times were changing; the courts continued to have a hand in shaping the mental health world.

The legal assault on psychiatry. Within a few short years, civil rights lawyers began to test the legal limits of the system of psychiatric hospitalization. Bruce Ennis, a leading attorney in the field, attacked involuntary hospitalization. His dramatically entitled book *Prisoners of Psychiatry* (Ennis, 1972) described his experiences in litigating on behalf of mental patients. Ennis claimed that a large number of individuals were confined without sufficient reason, were deprived of their rights while in institutions, and were subject to penalties and stigmatization upon release. His case studies are reminiscent of Mrs. Packard's almost a hundred years before.

Lawyers found psychiatrists were hard put to justify their opinions concerning the necessity for confinement. Scheff (1966) found that fully 100 percent of those examined by psychiatrists to determine commitability under the law were found commitable, whether or not there was evidence in their behavior that met statutory criteria of dangerousness to self or others. Psychiatric interviews lasted an average of 9 minutes; court hearings, in which the judge generally concurred with whatever psychiatric opinion was expressed, lasted no longer. Sometimes they were not held at all.

Attorneys developed methods of attacking psychiatric testimony. Ziskin (1974), writing for an audience of lawyers, carefully described the advantages and limits of scientific method in psychiatry and psychology, and explained the psychometric concepts of reliability and validity. Pointing out that information on the reliability and validity of clinical judgments made by individual practitioners was unknown, he showed how, on cross-examination, an attorney could take advantage of the difficulty: "Thus the process of clinical judgment appears to rest upon some process that may be mystical or perhaps art, but clearly is not science" (p.108).

Ennis and Siegel (1973) present interesting ideas and examples of cross-examination to show how difficult it may be for expert testimony by psychiatrists to stand up against rigorous cross-examination. (An earlier generation of attorneys were familiar with some of the techniques, as the transcript of Mrs. Packard's trial reveals [Packard (1875) 1973, Vol 2, p.31]). Attorneys found they could get clients out of hospitals, help them in commitment proceedings, and influence the courts. As we shall see, the courts' emphasis on restoring due process rights in civil as well as criminal commitments have made it more difficult to hospitalize, and to retain patients in the hospital. The legal decisions contributed toward deinstitutionalization and the necessity for community based care.

A mental patient's Bill of Rights. Step by step, federal judges enunciated the basic rights of patients. Although the specific order by a special three-judge panel in *Lessard* v *Schmidt* (1972) was vacated and remanded because of technical inadequacies (1974), its analysis of the issues of commitment and freedom was very influential. Miss Lessard was arrested by two police officers who filled out an emergency detention form. Three days later, a county court issued an order permitting her confinement for another ten days. Her detention was extended several more times until at a hearing, she was committed for thirty days by a judge who found her to be mentally ill. The thirty day commitment was extended one month, each month, until the suit reached the three-judge panel of the federal court to hear the constitutional claim. A class action suit alleged that she, and all others held involuntarily under provisions of the Wisconsin involuntary commitment statute, were denied due process of law.

The Circuit Court Judge placed the "fundamental liberty to go unimpeded about his or her affairs" very high in the value hierarchy, stating that society can deprive a person of that liberty only when it has a compelling interest in doing so. In criminal cases, one is deprived of liberty under the police power of the state, (the power to protect society against anti-social actions), but that power is tempered by "stringent procedural safeguards" to protect against arbitrary arrest or conviction. While the same fundamental liberty is at stake in civil commitment, the same due process safeguards have not been assured. The Court noted that no law would permit confinement of an individual on the basis that there was a high probability that the person would commit a crime in the future. However, a psychiatrist's recommendation for commitment is just such a prediction. Acceptance of the recommendation is justified on the grounds that there will be potential benefit to the person confined to a mental hospital.

The Court's decision provided a brief review of common law standards for involuntary confinement. In colonial days, even after the development of institutions, only those who were clearly deranged and violent were confined. Based on a court decision in a challenge to commitment brought in 1845, dangerousness to self was added as a criterion upon which to base commitment, an extension of English law principle that the state had a responsibility to care for the property of lunatics. If the state was responsible for the property of lunatics, why not for their persons?

Given that mental hospitals developed in the early nineteenth century on the premise that mental disorder was treatable, the confinement of the mentally incapacitated was viewed as a humanitarian act. Despite Mrs. Packard's successful efforts to introduce greater safeguards into the commitment procedure, after World War II, as Kittrie (1971) pointed out, the common law requirement of dangerousness shifted to include broad manifestations of "mental illness." The change of standard was accompanied by a relaxation of procedure, and a search for simpler and less traumatic means to bring help to individuals in need of help.

Noting the distinct relaxation of due process standards for involuntary incarceration, the Lessard Court was concerned that individuals receive the worst of two worlds: they receive neither adequate care, nor the protection of their rights. Considering the loss of numerous civil rights by virtue of civil commitment, the stigma associated with confinement to a mental institution, and a potentially higher mortality rate among those institutionalized, the Court stated that civil commitment was at least as damaging to the individual as conviction of a criminal offense. It therefore argued that the burdens on the state to justify commitment must be correspondingly high.

The Lessard Court then laid out what Brooks (1974) termed a potential bill of rights for mental patients. First, it insisted that the standard for commitment be interpreted to include a finding of "imminent danger to one self or others" based upon some "recent overt act, attempt or threat to do substantial harm to oneself or another." Vaguer standards of mental illness that do not include the requirement of such a finding would be disallowed as a basis for involuntary commitment.

The court also held that the standard of proof must be stringent, requiring "that the state must prove beyond a reasonable doubt all facts necessary to show that an individual is mentally ill and dangerous." In other words, it required the same standard of proof that is required when a defendant is deprived of liberty in a criminal proceeding. The Supreme Court has not followed that requirement (see *Addington* v *State of Texas*, 1979) for commitment of mental patients.

In addition the court indicated its belief that no one should be held for more than 48 hours on an emergency detention without a finding of probable cause at a preliminary hearing that a person is in need of commitment. A full hearing must be held as quickly as is feasible, generally within 10 to 14 days—sufficient time for necessary examinations to be conducted. The hearing must be scheduled well enough in advance to give the patient time to prepare, and the notice must include not only time, place, and date, but also the basis for detention, notice of the right to a jury trial, the standard upon which the patient may be detained, the names of examining physicians and prospective witnesses testifying in favor of the patient's commitment, and the substance of their proposed testimony. Moreover the right to counsel in such hearings was reaffirmed, as was the right of counsel to all reports introduced into the hearing. The court further affirmed that individuals should be afforded the equivalent of the privilege against self-incrimination; that is, the patient should be informed that he or she is to be examined with respect to his or her mental condition, any statements that are made may be the basis for commitment, and the patient does not have to speak to the psychiatrist. Furthermore, the court urged strict adherence to rules of evidence applicable in other proceedings in which an individual's liberty is at stake. Thus hearsay evidence (generally out-of-court statements, not given under oath, and not subject to cross-examination, introduced in proof of a point at issue) would be barred, except as such evidence is allowed by recognized exceptions to the hearsay rule.

The *Lessard* decision was important because it articulated patient rights in commitment procedures. Later cases (e.g., *Bartley* v *Kremens*, 1975) extended due process protections to children who were hospitalized on request of their parents. The U.S. Supreme Court, however, found a limit to legal intrusion into a parent's rights and duties to care for a child and limited the applicability of due process protections in that situation (*Parham* v *J.L. and J.R.*, 1979). Nonetheless, when taken together with decisions requiring treatment in the least restrictive alternative, it was clear that, at least from a formal legal viewpoint, the courts were going to examine very carefully procedures that arbitrarily incarcerated.

The least restrictive alternative. The attack on involuntary commitment made it more difficult to hospitalize patients. However, court decisions have also influenced the nature of the treatment situation for patients who are confined. Legal intervention has been in support of two propositions. One, that the patient has a right to treatment in the least restrictive alternative suitable for that patient's needs; and two, that the patient has a constitutional right to treatment.

The concept of the least restrictive alternative was enunciated in the case of *Lake* v *Cameron* (1966). Mrs. Lake, a sixty-year-old woman, was eventually committed to St. Elizabeth's Hospital after a policeman found her wandering about the city. She was not dangerous to others, and would not intentionally harm herself, but she was prone to "wandering away and being exposed at night or anytime that she is out." Mrs. Lake's *habeas corpus* petition failed. The lower court found she was dangerous to herself because she was not competent to care for herself. The court recognized that she might be entitled to release from St. Elizabeth's if another facility was available. Mrs. Lake appealed.

In the interim, a new District of Columbia statute allowed a trial court to order hospitalization as necessary, or to order "any other course of treatment" that the court believed would be in the best interests of the person and the public. In reviewing Mrs. Lake's case, Judge Bazelon said that in order to protect the interests of the individual and the public, a full spectrum of services, including outpatient or foster care, halfway houses, day hospitals, nursing homes, and other therapy facilities were all appropriate. Saying that the deprivation of liberty should not exceed what was necessary to protect an individual, he remanded the case asking the trial court to inquire into available alternatives for Mrs. Lake. He suggested, among other alternatives, one as minimally restrictive as requiring her to carry an identification card so police could take her home if she wandered. Although he asked the trial court to seek alternatives, he wisely refused to state what would happen if no available alternative was found.

It is a sad postscript that no suitable alternative was found. Mrs. Lake spent the last five years of her life in St. Elizabeth's, where she died, having received no visitors at all in her last year. In the absence of alternative facilities, the decision was ignored by Washington, D.C., judges (Brooks, 1974). It was not until a few years later that judges began ordering treatment facilities.

The concept of the least restrictive alternative was employed in *Covington* v *Harris* 1969). Covington, within a year after having served fourteen years for second-degree murder, was again charged with murder. Found incompetent to stand trial, he was committed to St. Elizabeth's, where seven years later, after a civil commitment, the murder charges were dropped. For years, Covington was a model patient in a maximum security ward. His psychiatrist recommended a transfer to a less secure service. When the institution's superintendent vetoed the transfer, Covington filed a writ of *habeas corpus*. At the trial, his physician changed his mind. However, the court said that a maximum security facility was not normally contemplated for civilly committed patients. Its extreme security entailed extraordinary deprivations of liberty and dignity, making it penitentiary-like, even if some treatment was provided. The court held that the principle of the least restrictive alternative held for dispositions made within a mental hospital, thus extending a right grounded in legal principles to the management of patients within an institution.

Another federal court (*Welsch* v *Likins*, 1974), citing other authorities, held that there is a constitutional duty on the part of institutional officials to explore and to provide for non-criminals the least stringent, practicable alternative to confinement. In this class action suit on behalf of residents in Minnesota state schools for the retarded, the decision held that options ranging from custody of a friend to placement within private institutions were all acceptable alternatives.

Although the judge agreed that state officials had made a good faith effort to provide alternatives, and were stymied by lack of funds and by legislative inaction, the court had extensive powers to order remedies to protect constitutional rights. The court could order the state officials to allocate resources, even though that is normally a legislative prerogative. The state could close the institution and not violate citizens rights, but the state could not confine without providing proper treatment. The judge stated his intent to monitor the efforts of institutional officials to correct conditions that violated patients' constitutional rights.

A federal court eventually ordered Washington, D.C., and officials of the federal government agency responsible for operating St. Elizabeth's Hospital to submit a plan to correct deficiencies in the provision of individualized treatment for patients civilly committed to that hospital (*Dixon* v *Weinberger*, 1975). The decision did *not* deal with a constitutional right. It was based on a District of Columbia statute that promised to provide psychiatric care and treatment to committed patients. The 1964 statute was construed to mean that patients confined in St. Elizabeth's Hospital were entitled to receive "suitable care and treatment under the least restrictive conditions as such conditions are required in an individual case . . ." (p.979).

Mr. Dixon, a 65-year-old voluntary patient, had been transferred to St. Elizabeth's from a general hospital because he had been confused, disoriented, and depressed. He spent the next twelve years in the hospital. During the next eight years after that, he lived in a foster home, returning to the hospital from time to time for treatment of physical illnesses. When he returned to the hospital in October 1972, he said he wanted to return to a good foster home as soon as possible. Mr. Dixon, a gentle, intelligent, sensitive man, by then confined to a wheel chair, was repeatedly recommended for placement in a home suitable for his needs. No action was taken. Mr. Dixon agreed to have the Mental Health Law Project, a public interest law firm, represent him. A suit was filed on his behalf. Within a few months, he was placed in a room and board facility in Washington, D.C.

Two social workers, one from the Mental Health Law Project, visited him in the board and care home. It was July 5, 1975, in the middle of a hot Washington, D.C., summer. They described their observations in testimony to a Senate Subcommittee:

> The conditions which we found at this facility or which Mr. Dixon told us about, were unconscionable. Mr. Dixon's sleeping room was about halfway below ground level. . . . The only windows in the room . . . were also closed and had a plate glass window in front of them making them difficult if not impossible for Mr. Dixon to open. They appeared to be painted shut. There

was no fan or air conditioner in the room, and although it was only 10 A.M., the room was already hot and stuffy. . . .

Mr. Dixon did not have a phone in his room. . . . There was no buzzer. We do not know how he would have contacted anyone if there was a fire or other emergency.

. . . Mr. Dixon had not been served any breakfast although he had been out of bed since 7 A.M. He stated that mealtimes were usually irregular and that sometimes he would get so hungry waiting for lunch he would ask a roomer to buy him sandwich meat and bread.

He could remember having only one glass of milk during his whole stay at the facility, which lasted six weeks, and virtually no fresh fruit. (U.S. Senate Subcommittee on Long Term Care, 1976, p.715)

Mr. Dixon returned to St. Elizabeth's following the July 5th visit, and eventually was placed in a suitable home. His case, while important in the legal development of the concept of the right to treatment in the most appropriate and least restrictive alternative, provides another lesson. Although the judge's order required an outline of a plan to be submitted within forty-five days, it took more than four years for a final plan to be formulated, and that plan is not to be implemented until December 31, 1981, a full six years after the decision was rendered. His case demonstrates a limitation of court-ordered change, a limitation discussed below.

The concept of the least restrictive alternative is defined in judicial orders requiring mental health officials to find or create settings which will allow patients to move from:

1. more to less structured living
2. larger to smaller facilities
3. larger to smaller living units
4. group to individual residences
5. places segregated from the community to places integrated with community living and programming, and
6. dependent to independent living.

(Comptroller General of the U.S., 1977, p.16)

The courts are saying that mental health officials must find or create such alternatives facilities, and seek funds or reallocate existing resources to provide for them. The courts are threatening to force compliance by issuing detailed orders backed by the court's coercive powers. The concept of the least restrictive alternative has led to little legal controversy, but in some of the decisions the concept of a constitutional right to treatment is linked to the least restrictive alternative. The concept of a constitutional right to treatment has generated more legal controversy because it is not a right spelled out explicitly in the Constitution, and would have to be inferred from other provisions and interpretations of those. It is also controversial because courts have vast powers to order remedial measures to correct constitutional violations, as we have seen in the school desegregation cases. If a constitutional right to treatment was established, the courts would have a firm basis everywhere for ordering far-reaching reforms.

The right to treatment. The concept of a right to treatment was developed by Birnbaum (1960), a lawyer and a psychiatrist. He stated the basic argument that if patients were not in the hospital for punishment, they were there to be helped, and if they were to be helped rather than warehoused, they had a right to treatment. Judge David Bazelon, a leading figure in the field, responsible for many important mental health decisions, gave formal recognition to the right-to-treatment concept in *Rouse* v *Cameron* (1966).

Rouse was found not guilty for reasons of insanity of carrying a concealed weapon, and was committed to St. Elizabeth's Hospital. He argued that he should either be set free or receive adequate treatment. The court agreed with him. For the first time ever, the decision mentioned a constitutional right to treatment. However, in a technical legal sense, its holding was based on an interpretation of the same District of Columbia statute used in the other cases. The statute promised every patient, according to Judge Bazelon's interpretation, humane care and medical treatment in accord with the highest standards accepted in medical practice, and as rapidly as possible despite shortages of staff or funds. A patient committed to a public hospital must have treatment appropriate to the individual's needs. If the individual did not receive such treatment, the state was violating individual rights and the individual should be released.

The demand that the patient receive treatment that was judicially determined to be adequate, and the assertion that lack of resources was not a good enough reason to deny an individual the right to treatment, was bold. However, the definition of adequate treatment was unclear, and in practice, the decision was apparently ignored by other judges and psychiatrists. In St. Elizabeth's, patients continued to receive tranquilizers as their major therapy, and they saw their doctors no more often than before. The doctors continued to rely on nurses and attendants reports to evaluate patients' conditions (Broderick, 1971).

A constitutional right to treatment was asserted a few years later in *Wyatt* v *Stickney* (1972), affirmed *sub nom. Wyatt* v *Aderholt* (1974).[4] Building on previous decisions, Judge Frank Johnson said:

> When patients are so committed for treatment purposes they unquestionably have a constitutional right to receive such individual treatment as will give each of them a realistic opportunity to be cured or to improve his or her mental condition. . . . Adequate effective treatment is constitutionally required because, absent treatment, the hospital is transformed into a penitentiary where one could be held indefinitely for no convicted offense. (*Wyatt* v *Stickney*, pp.781, 784)

Having found constitutional violations in two Alabama state hospitals, the court gave authorities six months to raise the level of care to the constitutionally required minimum. The class action was later enlarged to include patients in a state school for the retarded. Six months later, dissatisfied with the adequacy of the

4. As an interesting sidelight, we may note that the Wyatt case was initiated when cuts in the Alabama cigarette tax were reflected in cuts in the Mental Health Department budget. The Mental Health Department intended to fire 99 Bryce Hospital employees. The original complaint was filed by patients and employees jointly arguing patients wouldn't be able to get any treatment if the employees were fired. Recall that Goldman (1977) has suggested that patients and employees band together to assert their common interests against scarcity. The complaint was amended to a focus on patient care after an informal conference with the District Court Judge, who indicated that state employees could find relief through the state courts, but he was very concerned about the care of patients (Note Case, 1975).

treatment program implemented in that time, Judge Johnson ordered a hearing, receiving expert testimony in order to promulgate constitutionally adequate treatment standards. Experts representing the American Orthopsychiatric Association, the American Psychological Association, the American Civil Liberties Union, and the American Association on Mental Deficiency testified at the 1972 hearing. A set of standards for care and treatment emerged. These are worth citing in some detail since they indicate the changes necessary to meet constitutional standards, and they give some ideas of the costs.

To achieve a humane psychological and physical environment, the court ordered:

1. Patients have a right to privacy and dignity.

2. Patients have a right to the least restrictive conditions necessary to achieve the purpose of commitment.

3. No person shall be deemed incompetent to manage his affairs, to contract, to hold professional, or occupational or vehicle or operators' licenses, to marry and obtain a divorce, to register and vote, or to make a will *solely* by reason of his admission or commitment to the hospital.

4. Patients shall have the same rights to visitation and telephone communication as patients at other public hospitals [specific conditions of exception noted] . . . unrestricted right to visitation with attorneys and with private physicians and other health professionals.

5. Patients shall have an unrestricted right to send sealed mail . . . unrestricted right to receive sealed mail from their attorneys [other specified groups] . . . right to receive sealed mail from others [specific conditions of exception noted].

6. Patients shall have a right to be free from unnecessary or excessive medication. . . .

7. Patients have a right to be free from physical restraint and isolation, except for emergency situations [specific conditions noted].

8. Patients shall have a right not to be subjected to experi-

mental research without the express and informed consent of the patient. . . .

9. Patients have a right not to be subjected to treatment procedures such as lobotomy, electro-convulsive treatment, adversive reinforcement conditioning, or other unusual or hazardous treatment procedures without their express and informed consent after consultation with counsel or interested party of the patient's choice.

10. Patients have a right to prompt and adequate medical treatment for any physical ailments.

11. Patients have a right to wear their own clothes and to keep and use their own personal possessions. . . .

12. The hospital has an obligation to supply an adequate allowance of clothing to any patients who do not have suitable clothing of their own. Patients shall have the opportunity to select from various types of neat, clean, and seasonable clothing. Such clothing shall be considered the patient's throughout his stay in the hospital.

13. . . . provision for the laundering of patient clothing.

14. . . . the right to regular physical exercise. . . .

15. . . . right to be outdoors. . . .

16. The right of religious worship. . . .

17. . . . with adequate supervision, suitable opportunities for the patient's interaction with members of the opposite sex.

18. The following rules shall govern patient labor:
   A. Hospital Maintenance
      No patient shall be required to perform labor. . . . Privileges or release shall not be conditioned upon the performance of labor. . . . Patients may voluntarily engage in such labor if the labor is compensated in accordance with minimum wage laws. . . . (*Wyatt* v *Stickney*, pp.379–81)

The statement went on to define *therapeutic tasks* and *therapeutic labor*, permitting patients to do personal housekeeping (e.g., making one's own bed); did not allow the hospital to apply payments made to patients to the costs of care; specified adequate physical facilities and nutritional standards. It went on to specify the numbers and qualifications of staff in ratio to the number of patients. The Court order required that mental health professional staff meet all licensing and certification requirements for those engaged in private practice in Alabama, and orientation and in-service training for non-professional staff. Further it required that each nonprofessional staff member be directly supervised by a qualified mental health professional. The Court order listed a roster of 207.5 professional and nonprofessional full time staff per 250 patients including at least two psychiatrists who had completed three years of residency in psychiatry, four registered M.D.s, one Ph.D.-level psychologist with a degree from an accredited program, two M.S.W.s from accredited programs, twelve R.N.s, a vocational rehabilitation counselor, and sundry other aides, mental health workers, and clerical and support personnel. A similar and detailed staffing plan was specified for the Partlow Institution for the Retarded.

Beyond the staffing pattern, the court ordered that each patient have a detailed treatment plan, to be developed and implemented within five days of admission. The treatment plan must include a specification of the problem, statement of the least restrictive treatment conditions necessary, a time table for the attainment of treatment goals, a rationale for the program and specification of staff responsibility, criteria for release or discharge, and an individualized post-hospital plan. A case manager is required to supervise implementation of the treatment plan; detailed records are specified and special treatment and educational and recreational programs are required for children and young adults. Moreover, the court order stated that "the Mental Health Board and its agents have an affirmative duty to provide adequate transitional treatment and care for all patients released after a period of involuntary confinement" (*Wyatt* v *Stickney*, p.386).

As Stone (1975) points out, the court order in *Wyatt* v *Stickney* was designed to improve conditions in institutions that Stone described as Augean Stables in a state (Alabama) not noted for its generosity in its expenditures for the health and welfare of its citizens. Judge Johnson's order in *Wyatt* v *Stickney* was not based solely on the recommendations of professional experts. Cases litigated in the few years preceding established legal precedents for many of his requirements. Patients' rights within the hospital, the right to refuse treatment, and the right to be paid for patient labor directed toward hospital maintenance had all been litigated and won. The requirement that patient labor be compensated at at least minimum wage standards added to the financial costs of those institutions that relied on patient labor to minimize their personnel costs. (Summations of these cases and the issues they pose may be found in a variety of sources; for example, Ennis & Siegel, 1973; Brooks, 1974; and Stone, 1975; 1977.) Moreover, faced with court orders to expend vast sums on patient care, the move to release patients into the community may well have been accelerated. Stone (1977) claims:

> However, along with other similar developments, these lawsuits have hastened the precipitous discharge of thousands of patients from hospitals across the country. This process of rapid de-institutionalization has occurred without provision of adequate aftercare or alternative treatment facilities.
> The inescapable problem is that legally the right to treatment exists only when the state assumes responsibility for confining the patient. Thus the state can control the escalating costs of providing the right to treatment by rejecting the responsibility of confining patients. (p.276)

Stone is pessimistic about the impact of such right to treatment litigation because experience has shown that not very much happens. Stone states that there has been so little change that in an Ohio and a New York case the plaintiffs requested the courts hold the physicians and state officials in contempt of court (*Davis* v *Watkins*, 1974; *NYARC* v *Rockefeller*, 1973). The problems that are presented are important, and I shall discuss them in some detail later. They not only reveal how the system of mental health care is intimately tied into our whole political structure, but they also illuminate the problems of changing a complex social organization.

One more recent case, *O'Connor* v *Donaldson* (1975), has produced an intriguing result. This case reached the U.S. Supreme Court. Kenneth Donaldson, now 71 years old, was civilly committed to a Florida State Hospital in 1957 (when he was 47) o1 petition of his parents who were concerned about his mental state. Over the years he had repeatedly, but unsuccessfully, demanded his release on the grounds that he was not dangerous or insane.

His repeated requests for judicial relief were routinely denied. For whatever reason, Dr. J. B. O'Connor, Superintendent of the Florida hospital, blocked Donaldson's release each time. On one occasion, an organization that sponsored halfway houses offered to accept him and see that he received outpatient care. A family friend offered to provide him with living accommodations and appropriate supervision if Donaldson was released in his care. Dr. O'Connor repeatedly rejected the offers. During this time, Donaldson received little or no treatment. In fact, it was not disputed that Donaldson spoke to his doctor for a total of about two hours over a period of more than eight years. Donaldson told the U.S. Senate Subcommittee on Long Term Care (1976):

> I lost hundreds of friends who died from abuse. . . . I lived to tell the story. . . . Because of my belief in Christian Science, medication was not forced upon me . . . the treatment consists almost entirely of tranquilizer drugs. . . . An average doctor's call will last less than two minutes. . . . *Some patients went as much as 4 years, that I know of, without seeing a doctor, and some of them were on medication all that time.* . . . There was one doctor for 1300 men. He was licensed by the State of Florida only as an obstetrician. . . . People deteriorate physically when they are in confinement—even the young people. But many of the older people just gave up and they were not fit really to return to society. . . . I probably have brushed shoulders with 10,000 people on the various wards, coming and going and I actually know of only three that were schizophrenic during that time, who really needed some kind of care, who were afraid to go out in the free world. But the rest of them were not different than you and I are, except that they have been beaten down. That is all. (pp.713–74)

Superintendent O'Connor retired in 1971, and shortly afterwards, the staff discharged Donaldson. He thereupon brought suit for damages against Dr. O'Connor and other state hospital physicians, alleging that the defendants had intentionally and maliciously deprived him of his constitutional right to liberty. After a four-day jury trial, Donaldson won a verdict assessing compensatory and punitive damages in the amount of $38,500 against O'Connor and another staff physician. O'Connor lost an appeal in the Federal Circuit Court, and he carried the appeal to the U.S. Supreme Court.

The U.S. Supreme Court, in a carefully worded decision, said that it had no need to deal with the issue of whether there was a constitutional right to treatment upon compulsory confinement, or whether the State could compulsorily confine a nondangerous mentally ill individual for purposes of treatment. It did, however, say that the case did deal with the constitutional right to liberty. Since the jury had found that Donaldson was not dangerous to himself or others, and that if mentally ill he had not had treatment, the Court felt there was no reason to review those rationales for confining someone. Further, the Court reviewed several other possible reasons for confining Donaldson and rejected those. Even if his original confinement was valid, that fact alone did not justify continued confinement. A diagnosis of mental illness is not sufficient to justify continuing confinement. Confining someone to improve their condition of living is impermissible. Confining someone simply because the individual is different is certainly ruled out. The U.S. Supreme Court said:

> In short, a State cannot constitutionally confine without more a nondangerous individual who is capable of surviving safely in freedom by himself or with the help of willing and responsible family members or friends. *O'Connor v Donaldson*, (p.576)

The decision did not establish a constitutional right to treatment. On the contrary, the Supreme Court deliberately avoided dealing with that critical question. Chief Justice Burger took the trouble to write a concurring opinion, in which he said:

> In sum, I cannot accept the reasoning of the Court of Appeals and can discern no other basis for equating an involuntarily committed mental patient's unquestioned constitutional right not to be confined without due process of law with a constitutional right to treatment. Given the present state of medical knowledge regarding abnormal human behavior and its treatment, few things would be more fraught with peril than to irrevocably condition a State's power to protect the mentally ill upon the providing of "such treatment as will give (them) a realistic opportunity to be cured." Nor can I accept the theory that a State may lawfully confine an individual thought to need treatment and justify that deprivation of liberty solely by providing some treatment. Our

concepts of due process would not tolerate such a "tradeoff." Because the Court of Appeals analysis could be read as authorizing those results, it should not be followed. (pp.587–88)

The U.S. Supreme Court upheld the basic decision that Donaldson had been deprived of his civil right by O'Connor, and was entitled to damages. For other technical reasons, the case was sent back to the Court of Appeals for review of the award. Eventually, the Court of Appeals awarded Donaldson $20,000, and so far his day in court has resulted in a happier ending than many of the rest. Donaldson has since published a book detailing his experiences (Donaldson, 1976). He evidently has a good job in a hotel, and is living among friends.

The Supreme Court's decision seems to provide further legal support for the community based treatment of nondangerous individuals, and it seems to add to the general assault on involuntary commitment. Although there is no evidence on the point, I would expect that the possibility of being sued personally for damages related to the involuntary confinement of patients would have some effect on the willingness of hospital authorities to certify that individuals are in need of continued confinement.[5] However, Chief Justice Burger in his concurring opinion was careful to point out there are many precedents for hospitalization, including the protection of society (police power) and the care of those unable to care for themselves (parens patriae).

Chief Justice Burger's opinion seems to say that it is not such a bad thing to confine people who are chronically unable to care for themselves. So far, his opinion does not seem to have set off a new wave of custodial confinements. It may be another illustration that the dynamics of care proceed in their own way despite what the courts say. As I pointed out in earlier chapters, states have considerable financial incentive to continue to deinstitutionalize. It is not likely that we will soon return to the large custodial institutions of the past, despite whatever support might be found in the Court's ruling. While cases based on the right to

5. The liability of physicians in a commitment proceeding is far from a new legal concept. Ordronaux (1878) pointed out in his review of New York State insanity laws that physicians signing a certificate maliciously, or without probable cause, or without having carefully conducted their own inquiries are subject to suit. Such suits evidently have not been brought very often in recent times.

treatment have slowed down, litigants have found enough basis in state and federal statutes to move against institutions to reform them (e.g. *Halderman* v *Pennhurst State School and Hospital,* 1978). As the Circuit Court in *Halderman* recognized, federal policy still supports deinstitutionalization, and the courts had, so far, interpreted the law in support of cleaning up the worst of our institutional messes, and in favor of the establishment of community based facilities. *Halderman* v *Pennhurst State School and Hospital* was reviewed by the U.S. Supreme Court in April 1981. The finding of the Circuit Court that federal legislation provided an affirmative duty on the institution to provide treatment in the least restrictive alternative was reversed, and remanded for further consideration. The Supreme Court's decision was based on an interpretation of the significance of one section of one federal statute (§6010 of the Developmentally Disabled Assistance and Bill of Rights Act of 1975, 42 U.S.C. §§ 6000 et seq). The decision, however, revealed the present Court's disinclination to pursue either the right to treatment concept or the notion that patients have a right to treatment in the least restrictive alternative.[6]

Justice Rehnquist's decision may be salutory in one respect. It delicately exposes congressional hypocrisy in "mandating" far reaching changes for others to accomplish without, at the same time, providing federal funds to accomplish the change. The decision is lacking in moral tone in that there is little discussion of the reasons for the action against the institution in the first place. Justice Rehnquist limits his discussion to the bland sentence summarizing the findings of the trial court: "Its findings of fact are undisputed: Conditions at Pennhurst are not only dangerous, with the residents often physically abused or drugged by staff members, but inadequate for the "habilitation" of the retarded. Indeed the court found that the physical, intellectual and emotional skills of some residents have deteriorated at Pennhurst" (pp.4364–65). Those findings of fact might have resulted in a minimum statement

6. Woodward and Armstrong (1979) claim that Chief Justice Burger and Judge David Bazelon were long-time antagonists when both served on the District of Columbia Circuit Court, on the concepts of the right to treatment and the least restrictive alternative. Given the growing conservative bent of the Supreme Court, the future of those concepts at the level of the Supreme Court, and in lower federal courts, to the degree they follow the Supreme Court's lead, is not bright.

of concern that there is an urgent need to avoid and improve such conditions, or that their existence violates our collective conscience, but no such expression of moral sentiment is found in Mr. Rehnquist's technically oriented legal opinion. Mr. Justice White, writing in dissent, was more explicit that there is a need to improve outrageous conditions in institutions.

Trial courts, dealing with the direct human exhibits of institutional failures, may be more sensitive to the humane issues than the paper oriented appellate courts. Courts have ordered mental hospitals and institutions for the retarded to make expensive changes. Some state officials have tried to comply in good faith, within the limits of their resources. Others have simply discharged patients into the community and refused to take direct responsibility for them. Still others have ignored the courts or complied in minimal or token fashion, forcing further litigation. Judges have more and more taken to appointing monitors and special masters to oversee compliance. While the paper victories (Bradley & Clarke, 1976) look impressive, the law on the books is not the same as the law in action, and it is to a review of the law in action that we now turn.

Chapter 6

IMPLEMENTATION OF CHANGES THROUGH THE LAW
Success, Failures, and Limitations

At the risk of oversimplifying, we might say the legal theory of social and institutional change is summed up by the proposition that legislators and judges mandate change with the expectation that law abiding citizens will make every effort to comply. In general, those expectations are borne out. The mandates can be enforced by the vast coercive powers of the state when individuals violate them. While most laws are effective in some degree, not all laws achieve their goals. Each one may be thought of as an experiment in planned social change, and some experiments go awry. They are ineffective. They do not achieve their purposes. They partially achieve their purposes, but they have unfortunate side effects, or the resources allocated were simply insufficient to do the job, even if the methods could have attained the goals, as in the 1960's War on Poverty.

Even though legislatively or judically mandated change is legitimate, in the sense that the legislature in theory reflects the popular will, or that judges are delegated vast powers to interpret the laws and to fashion remedies when inequities are discovered, those affected by the laws do not always obey them. The laws may be ignored, or if not ignored then violated in spirit so that the outcome is different than its designers intended. Nowhere is the problem better revealed than when orders for change affect isolated, relatively autonomous institutions or where those affected by the law are dealing with relatively intractable social problems, and lack either the resources, the imagination, the will or the leadership to give life to cultural ideals which may be reflected in the statement of the law.

The order for change does not exist in isolation. It is necessarily shaped by the context in which it must be implemented. The order for change may conflict with other laws or administrative regulations posing dilemmas for those who must carry out contradictory mandates. The rhetoric of individual rights, or of rehabilitation, encounters the realities of security considerations in prisons. It is not unusual for the national legislature to mandate changes for local institutions, but then not to provide necessary funds. Public Law 94–142 mandates mainstreaming in the public schools, but the amount of federal funds thus far appropriated to support the programs falls far short of what was promised in the legislation. Sometimes an order fails to take into account the realities of dealing with difficult problems. The social technology for accomplishing rehabilitation may be too uncertain in its effects, or the best that can be accomplished may fall far short of what should be accomplished ideally. An order for change may conflict with deep-seated cultural values or prejudices, as in school desegregation orders requiring busing into the suburbs, or the busing of white children into black neighborhoods.

The order to change can be defeated by institutional defenses against mandated change. It can be subject to delay as further litigation is pursued in appeals or in new cases challenging a statute or interpretations of its provisions. And, of course, if anything is predictible about the judicial system it is that almost every action will be subject to delay and numerous postponements due to crowded calendars and the courtesies lawyers extend to each other so that all may work more or less at their convenience.

Orders can be circumvented, subverted, or even ignored. Officials can salami slice, taking minimal or token steps to comply, but avoiding coming to grips with the problem that legal action was meant to correct. Responsibility for implementing aspects of the required changes can be so diffuse that it is difficult to pin down exactly who is responsible for what. Top-level officials may say they want change, but the order may not reach line-level workers who simply continue doing what they have always done. Levine and Schweber-Koren (1976) accounted for sex discrimination in jury selection by the actions of female clerks who didn't send jury notices to women because they believed women would take advantage of a then-existing women's waiver, and wouldn't want to serve anyway. Attendants in hospitals, clerks, assistant principals in schools, corrections officers, houseparents, or welfare workers may not change in the absence of skilled and determined line leadership, which if available would show how change can and should be accomplished. The apparently simple matter of obtaining adequate information about the degree of compliance can result in delays, conflict, and further litigation.

The legal theory of mandated change does not fully take into account barriers to implementation inherent in social complexity. That the legal theory of change ends with the law on the books is demonstrated by the lack of evaluative mechanisms formally built into the law. There are, of course, many informal channels through which the effectiveness of existing law and the necessity for change are evaluated. But laws are not usually regarded as experiments whose results are to be systematically evaluated. Data accumulate, however, and it is to an examination of the results, both intended and unintended, of legally mandated change that we now turn.

Involuntary hospital admissions. One thrust of litigation and concomitant legislative change has been to make involuntary hospitalization subject to greater due process protections. Presumably it is now more difficult to hospitalize than it was before. What have been the effects on involuntary hospital admissions? In 1933 (Meyer, 1974), 90 percent of all first admissions to state and county hospitals were by court commitment, and only 5 percent were voluntary. By 1972, 54.3 percent were voluntary or nonprotesting admissions. The figures, however, may be deceptive. Miller (1976) believes that patients are offered a choice of accepting voluntary commitment or of becoming subject to a legal proceeding. Even a voluntarily admitted patient is not free to come and go as he or she chooses. The patient signs in for a period of time that may be renewable. The patient may be discharged only with the approval of hospital authorities, although in many states, the patient may request a hearing.

While sex makes only a small difference for the frequency of involuntary admissions (42 percent of female admissions; 47 percent of male admissions), race and education do make for important differences. Fewer whites (43.2 percent) than blacks (56.0 percent) and fewer of those with college educations (40.7 percent) than those with less than seventh-grade education (54.3 percent) are involuntary admissions. The effect is most pronounced for women with college educations—only 32.1 percent are involuntary admissions. Nonwhites with less than eighth-grade educations are most likely to be admitted involuntarily—71.2 percent of admissions are in that category.

Larger demographic differences are apparent in the figures of those committed as incompetent to stand trial. In general, such admissions are a small proportion of all admissions. Admissions for incompetency to stand trial are concentrated among males in the 18 to 24 age range. There are a negligible number among females in that age range, but 9.3 percent of all male admissions are for that reason. Race interacts with sex. Only 1.8 percent of white males aged 18–24 are committed as incompetent to stand trial, but 21.6 percent of all nonwhite male admissions are for that reason. Even controlling for differences in education, a difference emerges between whites and nonwhites. Only 1.4 percent of whites with less than seventh-grade educations are admitted as incompetent to stand trial, but 8.9 percent of all nonwhites with the same educational level are admitted as incompetent to stand trial. It is difficult to think of clinical correlates of the demographic data to rationalize the race differences (Meyer, 1974).

Meyer's findings were based on data cumulated nationally. Luckey and Berman (1979) studied a change in Nebraska's mental health law, made in 1976, to bring its procedures for involuntary commitment closer in line with the due process requirements laid down in many court decisions. The new law required "clear and convincing" proof (a higher standard than "preponderance," but less than "beyond a reasonable doubt") that a person is both mentally ill and dangerous to self and others, as manifested by recent acts, or is unable to provide for his or her own basic needs. The new law incorporated procedural changes—hearings, the right to independent professional evaluation, the right to an attorney, and a mandatory review within 60 days after commitment

actions. The new law's stricter criteria and more rigorous procedures should have resulted in a decline in involuntary admissions.

Indeed, a sophisticated time-series analysis did detect such a
decline shortly after the new law was passed, but within eighteen
months, the proportion of statewide involuntary admissions was
just as it was before the law was passed. Males were involuntarily
committed as often under the new law as under the old, although
the proportion of females declined. Younger people were more
likely to be committed under the new procedure than they were
under the old one. The less well-educated were more subject to
involuntary commitment than the better educated, although in
Nebraska no relationship was found with race.

Luckey and Berman concluded that the decrease was temporary because commitment boards, after an initial period of adjustment to the new law, were simply not implementing it as its
designers had intended. Making it more difficult to commit a
patient to the hospital didn't solve the problem of what to do with
a distressed individual, and his or her family, in the absence of
alternative facilities in the community to care for those in need.

Variability in the application of laws. Because commitment
laws vary state by state, we can expect variation on that account.
Miller (1976) reports that in 1970, proportions of involuntary
admissions ranged from 10 percent in Alaska to 90 percent in
Florida. Involuntary admissions ranged from 30 percent to 77
percent in states with more than 10,000 admissions a year. There
are equally wide variation in proportions of involuntary commitments county by county within a state where all courts are presumably operating with the same laws. Miller reports that the
proportion of involuntary admissions ranged from 32 percent to
95 percent in 58 counties in California. The odds of being found
competent in a competency proceeding ranged from zero (no
chance at all) to about 50 percent in different counties in Florida.

Broderick (1971) showed that practices among District of
Columbia federal court judges varied widely in how each handled
different aspects of commitment proceedings. Although many of
the leading decisions in patients rights suits were won in the
District of Columbia Appellate Court, there is no evidence of any
more consistency of practice, nor adherence to the rules in that

circuit than in any other.[1] Between 40 and 50 percent of petitions from St. Elizabeth's Hospital patients were not heard, nor did the court appoint an attorney for them. At the time, an administrative official in the court decided whether to grant a hearing. Petitions from patients were accompanied by informal recommendations from the hospital, and turndowns were justified on the grounds that petitioners were chronic filers. However, a follow up showed that only 9 percent of those turned down had had a hearing in the previous six months, and only 5 percent of all petitioners were repeaters.

Similar court-to-court variability was reported by Gupta (1971) for New York State. The 1964 revision of the New York Mental Hygiene Law established a Mental Health Information Service (MHIS) as a watchdog for patients' rights responsible to the Appelate Court in New York. New York State is divided into four judicial districts or departments. The Chief Judge in each department selects MHIS staff who are responsible for notifying patients of their rights, and their rights to a hearing. Whenever judicial commitment is involved, whether or not it is contested, MHIS provides an independent report for the court concerning relevant facts and available alternatives to hospitalization.

Mental patients may be heard in court in several different types of hearings (after initial emergency hospitalization; for continued commitment; habeas corpus, when a patient is not released). The rates of discharge after having received a hearing ranged from zero (no discharges at all) to 50 percent, and the rates varied unpredictibly from judicial department to department, and for type of hearing and in different years. It appears as if rather arbitrary considerations determine the rates of discharge.

There were wide variations in the number of cases seeking hearings. One upstate judicial department had a grand total of 7 hearings in 3 years, while there were 551, 798, and 805 hearings in the other 3 departments. Gupta (1971) attributes the difference to

1. It is far from clear that patients were benefited by reformers. At St. Elizabeth's, the mean waiting time in the institution for completed psychiatric examinations increased from 2.4 months in 1959 to 4.5 months by 1969. In 1964–67, prior to some of the important decisions, 80 percent of St. Elizabeth's patients waited *less* than 60 days for the psychiatric examination to be completed. In the 1967–69 period, 94 percent waited *more* than 60 days (Broderick, 1971).

variation in the staffing patterns. Downstate staffs are comprised largely of lawyers, while the upstate office was staffed by social workers. In essence, he reports variability, when ideally, if everyone enjoyed the equal protection of the law, the application of the law should be unvarying.

Luckey and Berman (1979) reported similar geographic variation in the application of a new Nebraska Mental Hygiene law. There was a significant decrease in involuntary commitments in rural counties with populations less than 14,000. Following the passage of the law, although the proportion of involuntary commitments dropped, with time they increased again. The increase in the rate of change of involuntary commitments after the law was passed was significant in counties with populations greater than 100,000, and nearly statistically significant in middle-size counties. Luckey and Berman attributed the differences in the application of the new law to the willingness and ability of county governments to bear the expense it entailed. Rural counties were less willing or less able to bear the expenditures for holding hearings and paying expert witnesses. Luckey and Berman speculate that tolerance for deviance may be as much a function of the costs of implementing formal social controls through mental health law as it is of other community attitudes. They also speculated that in rural counties, people who are potential patients simply go to jail instead.

Variations in the application of the law raise questions about how much the laws do afford equal protection, and how much individuals are subject to the vagaries of individual judges, local attitudes, the availability of funds and facilities, and a number of other practical matters not controlled by the law on the books. We cannot say whether the variation is greater or less in this area of the law than in any other, but because the control of deviance involves basic values, and because most of those who are involved in the process as potential patients are relatively powerless, the formal protections of law are all the more important, if we are to live up to the manifest cultural ideal which states that we are a society based on law, not on people. For the time being, we will pass over the implications for our understanding of the mental health system of these vagaries in the application of law.

Representation by an attorney is considered among the most

important of due-process safeguards. The Sixth Amendment to the Constitution guarantees the right to representation by counsel in criminal prosecutions where liberty is at stake. In *Gideon* v *Wainwright* (1963), the Supreme Court made it mandatory that all defendants in felony actions be represented by counsel, and at state expense if the individual was indigent. The Supreme Court has not passed on the precise issue as far as commitment is concerned, but the analogy seems obvious. In fact, in the last fifteen or twenty years, patients have had greater opportunities for representation with regard to hospitalization and release. Has representation by attorney had the desired effects?

Legal representation. Representation by counsel in commitment hearings makes a difference. Wenger and Fletcher (1969) reported a .94 correlation between presence of a counsel and likelihood of being released in a commitment hearing. Miller (1976) cites another study in which representation resulted in approximately one third of the cases being released or continued, where only 6.4 percent were released if no attorney represented the prospective patient at a commitment hearing. Kittrie (1971) cites other data in which public defenders report rates of dismissal in commitment hearings ranging from 15 percent to 70 percent.

Representatives of the MHIS in New York are not supposed to act as patient advocates. However, Gupta (1971) reports that in a series of 55 consecutive cases he observed in court, the MHIS representative seemed in favor of discharge in 18. The patient was discharged in 12 of those instances. The patients were committed in the other 6 cases. Only 1 of 37 other cases was discharged at these commitment hearings. Miller (1976) cites a California study which showed that even the presence of observers in court can make a difference. During a month that the California Mental Health Association sent observers into court, only 43 percent of cases were committed. In the previous month, when no observers were present, 76 percent were committed.

In addition to assisting patients in formal hearings, attorneys have been successful in negotiating out-of-court settlements for their clients. In the first three years of the operation of New York's MHIS, there was a statewide decline in the proportion of cases asking for a hearing from 8.0 percent to 4.6 percent, no small reduction in the state court workload when thousands are hospitalized each year. Gupta (1971) stated that at Bellevue Hospital in New York City, where the best records were kept, the proportion of requests for hearings on continued hospitalization that were *withdrawn* before getting to court increased from 44.7 percent to 64.0 percent over a four-year period. Of these cases where the requests for hearing were withdrawn, an average of 60 percent were settled by the psychiatrist discharging the patient. In the remaining instances, the patient accepted voluntary hospitalization.

Kittrie (1971) was only modestly pleased with these results. He saw further problems for the legal profession:

> These statistics by no means demonstrate that all those kept from being committed indeed were afflicted with no mental problems. They do indicate, however, that presence of counsel may guarantee more careful attention to the question of whether commitment is the appropriate social solution in a given case. (p.94)

Kittrie agrees that the function of attorneys generally became more and more ceremonial as the procedures became more informal and as courts and attorneys tended to accede to psychiatric opinion. He accepts that in order for due process safeguards to be meaningful, judge and counsel must be "taught to understand sociopsychological data and to assume a newly critical role for which they had not hitherto been prepared" (p.95). Judges, despite recent ligitation and publicity, still defer to psychiatric judgment. Albers and Pasewark (1974) reported that judges agreed with psychiatric recommendations 95 percent of the time, and although she reported a lower frequency of uncritical agreement, Hiday (1977) found judges agreed with psychiatric judgment even in the absence of substantiating evidence.

In his comment, Kittrie assumes that the problems which were uncovered were a function of a willingness on the part of members of the legal profession to accede to the expertise of psychiatrists. He seems to say that knowledge and reliance on adversarial process will be sufficient to solve the problems. While it is obvious that as a consequence of legal action, fewer patients are incarcerated involuntarily, and that a patient can enhance chances of discharge if represented, or even by threatening to ask for a hearing, if representation is available, it is not clear that patient rights will be preserved in the general run of cases.[2]

The training of judges and lawyers is only a part of the problem. Poythress (1978) reported an experiment in training court-appointed defense lawyers to use effective cross-examining techniques in commitment hearings that was an utter failure. The lawyers learned and understood the techniques but refused to use them in practice. Attorneys who were convinced their clients were disturbed and needed help were unwilling to argue very strenuously that their clients should not be committed. Moreover, the attorneys in the experiment were not convinced the judges wanted them to advocate very vigorously. (See also Warren, 1977, for a similar observation.) Both lawyers and judges felt that something had to be done for the patients.

Scheff (1966) had a somewhat more cynical view of the motives of lawyers and judges in commitment proceedings. He notes they can get in little political trouble for holding patients, but can get in a great deal of difficulty if a released patient commits a crime that comes to public notice. Reasoning that commitment for observation or for treatment can do little harm, and might do some good, Scheff argues that lawyers, judges, and psychiatrists are prone toward committing rather than releasing, especially in the absence of alternatives to outright release. Warren (1977) observed judges ignoring statutory criteria for commitment out of a felt necessity to protect against potential violence, to relieve families of burdens, to protect a seemingly helpless person, or to remove a nuisance from the streets.

The economics of public representation presents another problem. In a Texas court, a court-appointed attorney handled 40 cases in a single hearing. He admitted to an interviewer that he had had previous contact with only two of the cases, and that he was unprepared in all the rest. The 40 cases were disposed of by the judge in 75 minutes. The judge allowed the court appointed

2. Representation by public defenders in the juvenile courts, a post-*Gault* requirement to protect due process rights, may paradoxically have resulted in an *increased* frequency of commitment to juvenile institutions. Clarke and Koch (1980) found the participation of counsel was token and ceremonial rather than integral to fact finding.

attorney a fee of $10.00 per case, or a total of $400 for what could not have been two hours of professional legal work (Cohen, 1966). Kittrie (1971) states that in 22 states which then required counsel to be appointed at a patient's request, maximum fees ranged from $10.00 to $25.00. In other states, numerous cases are assigned to a single staff attorney of a legal aid society, or inexperienced private attorneys are appointed at random. Obviously, the best one can expect under these circumstances is superficial representation (Clarke & Koch, 1980). Similar slipshod practices, determined by necessity but bordering on the unethical, were noted by Hostica (1974) in his observational study of the application of summary process, the procedure for evicting tenants from rented apartments.

The President's Commission on Mental Health (1978b) endorsed the further development of advocacy systems to protect the mentally disabled, based on the report of its Task Panel on Legal and Ethical Issues. The Task Panel Report emphasized the advantages of advocacy but did not review its concrete results. Advocacy, with nothing more, will not accomplish its desired ends, and in fact one must question the ethics of advocacy which in substance leaves people no better off than they were before. Members of the legal profession have an ethical responsibility to review their own actions, just as do physicians and scientists. The responsibility of lawyers may even be greater, for the legal profession is at home in the courts, and can use coercive power. No other profession has the same access to this powerful instrument of social control. And self-evaluation is of paramount importance for judges, as they are responsible for overseeing the applications of the law. What has been their role?

Responsibilities of the judge. Judges, in the American legal system, have awesome responsibilities and vast powers. Their decisions make a difference for life, liberty, property, and the pursuit of happiness for those seeking redress or conflict resolution through the courts. But it is not only judges' decisions that are important. A judge sets the tone for the courtroom. It was a judge who observed and worked with the Texas attorney who handled forty cases in 75 minutes and it was the judge who authorized the payment of $400 for less than two hours of legal work (Cohen,

1966). It was the judges in Florida courtrooms who routinely denied Donaldson's petitions for release even though the hospital staff agreed he was not dangerous to himself or others. Donaldson was able to collect damages against O'Connor, but judges have immunity for their official actions on the bench. No Florida judge was a co-defendant in the case, although a layman might well feel the judge who failed to review Donaldson's petitions independently and thoroughly was guilty of negligence, in the common-sense meaning of that term.

The judge in *Bartley* v *Kremens* (1975) expressed the opinion that one did not need a jury trial in meeting due process requirements in commitment hearings for children since judges are well able to discern the facts, and make the decisions. Perhaps so, but it is not clear judges use those powers of discernment very carefully in the normal run of cases. Scheff (1966) reported that a substantial percentage of those committed as dangerous to self or others, based on a psychiatric recommendation, did not reveal overt signs of such dangerousness. Yet the courts uniformly supported the psychiatric recommendations. One of the attorneys that Poythress (1978) trained to cross-examine psychiatric experts claims a judge told him, off the record, that it wouldn't make any difference if he argued three minutes or three hours. The client was going to be committed anyway. Scheff believes that judges lean toward commitment on the assumption that treatment could do no harm, and to protect against the possibility that public criticism would result if a patient who was released then harmed someone else. Scheff believed that it was not only that judges agreed with psychiatric expert witnesses. He believed that judges also selected psychiatric experts who would provide the court with the opinions the court wanted.

Albers, Pasewark, and Smith (1976) studied the written petitions for 50 consecutive patients committed involuntarily to a state hospital. In that state, an affidavit must be filed containing evidence of mental illness. A court order is then issued and the individual is brought in for a short examination. The complainant, the prospective patient, his attorney if he has one, and the examining physicians appear for a hearing. The judge decides whether the patient is mentally ill and should be committed. In only five cases, or 10 percent of the 50 consecutive petitions, did the complainant provide an affidavit that the patient was a danger to himself or others. Yet in all fifty cases the examining physicians certified the person as dangerous, and the judge never looked at the evidence either for or against. Warren (1977) and Hiday (1977) reported a similar tendency of judges to disregard the evidence in arriving at decisions, in many cases.

Albers and Pasewark (1974) reported that judges agreed with psychiatric recommendations 95 percent of the time in 300 cases, with the median hearing time being 8 minutes. Scheff (1966) reported the hearings he observed lasted an average of 1.6 minutes, with the judge asking two or three perfunctory questions before committing the prospective patient. It is not that the evidence of mental illness was so overwhelmingly obvious. Scheff believed that in nearly 40 percent of the cases, the psychiatric examinations failed to establish mental illness according to the criteria judges claimed they were using. The psychiatric interviews themselves lasted an average of 9.2 minutes.

It was not only the psychiatrists who were hasty. Scheff observed 12 interviews of patients with guardians *ad litem* (lawyers who are appointed to represent the patients). In none of the twelve interviews did the guardians inform patients of their legal rights. According to Warren's observation (1977), judges and attorneys engaged in the equivalent of plea bargaining either in advance of a commitment hearing, or during it. Miller (1976) based on a review of a large number of studies concluded that the average time consumed in involuntary commitment hearings was under five minutes. The 16.5 minutes reported for New York cases with Mental Health Information Service personnel present was unusually long, although Hiday (1977) reported that commitment hearings lasted about that long in North Carolina courtrooms following passage of a new commitment law.

Considering what is at stake for the prospective patient, court hearings move very rapidly indeed. Chu and Trotter (1974) report that while 94 percent of all prisoners in federal prisons had terms of five years or less, 66 percent of all patients resident at St. Elizabeth's Hospital in Washington, D.C., in 1970 had been in the institution more than five years, and 53 percent more than ten years.

It is trite to say "It's the system," but in this case it *is* the system. While higher courts have been extending due process rights, the emphasis on more stringent procedure will not in and of itself result in better patient care, and it is not even clear that in the general run of cases, the emphasis really results in safeguarding patient rights. Justice Fortas, *In re Gault* (1967), faulted juvenile courts for not helping youth, and he ordered more stringent procedures to protect their legal rights. The history of the Packard laws however suggests that even when jury trials, using the stringent rules of criminal procedure, were required, judges and attorneys colluded to move the trials as quickly as possible to expedite hospitalization. In fact, Clarke and Koch (1980) report just such a collusion in juvenile court hearings after *Gault*, in which juveniles are represented by attorneys.

The emphasis on formal doctrine and upon ritually observing form while assuming that substance will thereby be protected represents a conceit of the paper-oriented legal system that the real world doesn't matter. While judges sometimes consider the hospital administration's convenience in reviewing the rationality of procedures (e.g., Justice Rehnquist's dissent in *Califano* v *Goldfarb*, 1977), we have not yet seen a like concern for the consequences of changing a system without first understanding how that system operates on a day-to-day level.

Gupta (1971) formulated a corollary of Parkinson's law for the work of the court. Whenever there is a heavy flow of work, without a concomitant increase in resources, the amount of time devoted to each unit is decreased. As an inference from that general proposition, the more the courts require the formalites of due process, without concomitant increases in resources, the more we can expect that each element of due process will be given more and more perfunctory attention. Scheff (1966) pointed out that guardians *ad litem* and psychiatrists, who are both paid low fees per capita, increase their rates by limiting the amount of time they spend with each client. The rule has applicability to all the players in the game. One can predict that as the requirements for due process intensify, we will see more and more compliance on paper, for the record, with less attention to each individual.

The requirements may result in more work for lawyers and for mental health workers attached to the courts, but whether the increased demand for their services will result in improved protection of the rights of the helpless, the repulsive, and the poor remains to be seen. None of the studies showing an increase in patient releases with legal representation have shown what happened to the patients who were released, or to their families. Judging from the Baxtrom patients discussed above, and from studies such as that by Tuckman and Lavell (1962) showing that patients discharged against medical advice from a psychiatric service did just as well as those receiving regular discharges, their release may not have had any harmful effects. Courts and laywers are not overly self-critical of their work, and they generally have no obligation to determine what happens to the people involved once the legal work has been completed. However, lawyers and judges have been important forces in institutional reform, and we turn now to an examination of the methods that have been employed and their outcomes.

Consequences of legal action for patient care. We have already noted that Mrs. Lake, the successful plaintiff in the landmark case of *Lake* v *Cameron* (see Chapter 5), was little benefited by her victory in court. Mr. Dixon, chief complainant in another landmark class action suit *Dixon* v *Weinberger* (1975), was first placed in a miserable boarding home, and then returned to the hospital at his own request. (He is now residing comfortably in a suitable home.) Since those were the outcomes for the principal plaintiffs in the class action suits, we can guess at the outcomes for others not so visibly represented. The problem of introducing change into complex social organizations cannot be underestimated. Nowhere is the complexity of the problem clearer than in follow-up efforts to implement changes consequent to court decisions asserting the right to treatment in the least restrictive alternative.

In *Wyatt* v *Stickney* (1971), Federal District Court Judge Frank Johnson found patients who were involuntarily committed to Alabama's state hospitals and state schools had a *constitutional* right to adequate treatment, and they were not receiving adequate treatment.[3] Mental health officials requested six months to

3. *Wyatt* v *Stickney* was based on a constitutional interpretation in which a right to treatment was derived from other constitutionally recognized rights. When a violation is based in the constitution, the judge has far-reaching powers to order

raise standards to the constitutionally required minimum. Judge Johnson granted the request, but required reports showing progress in implementing changes to meet constitutionally mandated standards (see Chapter 5).

Six months later, having received the institutions' reports, Judge Johnson concluded that defendants had failed to promulgate and implement a treatment program satisfying minimum medical and constitutional requisites. He thereupon ordered a further formal hearing in which plaintiffs, defendants, and *amici curiae* (friends of the court) would have the opportunity to submit statements of appropriate standards backed by expert witnesses who would testify in support of their proposals. A hearing was held early in 1972 in which the American Orthopsychiatric Association, the American Psychological Association, the American Civil Liberties Union, and the American Association of Mental Deficiency were all represented. Some of the foremost authorities on mental health in the United States expressed their views at this time. Following the hearing, Judge Johnson formulated the set of explicit standards referred to in Chapter 5, and ordered Alabama mental health officials to comply (*Wyatt* v *Stickney*, 1972).

Enforcement of judicial decisions is quite another matter. It is relatively simple to enforce an injunction prohibiting a specific, definable act through use of the court's contempt powers. It is also relatively straightforward to provide for an award of monetary damages, and to see to it that these are collected eventually. However, these traditional solutions have little relevance to an order designed to change a total institution.

An institution can adopt a variety of defenses against a court order. It can make a very small change, which meets the letter of

---

remedies even in the absence of other laws passed by a state legislature. A constitutionally based decision is important because of its great ramifications. The U.S. Supreme Court is the ultimate aribiter of constitutional rights, and as yet it has neither confirmed nor denied there is a constitutionally based right to treatment. Chief Justice Burger wrote a concurring opinion in *Donaldson* v *O'Connor* (see Chapter 5) in which he went out of his way to indicate that he at least was not favorably disposed to the concept. The *Halderman* case is important, for the Supreme Court's decision in that case may well have a critical impact on the future of institutional reform litigation, especially in those states where there is no statutory basis for a claim to appropriate care within an institution or in the community.

the court order, but which has little to do with the substance of
the complaint. A new form of abuse, not prohibited in the court
order, can replace the first one. Outsiders can be kept from
getting information, as the nineteenth century hospital superintendents did by barring visitors when they became the targets of
law suits (Caplan, 1969). The judge may not have the expertise to
judge the institution's claims, stated in technical language that
some action is necessary, or that one act is the equivalent of
another. It may be difficult to penetrate a bureaucracy to determine exactly how it works, to pin down responsibility for given
acts. Even a willing institutional administration may not have
sufficient control, or sufficient information to fix responsibility
within the organization. In many instances, hard, dirty jobs are
handled by line personnel who derive considerable de facto
power simply because they do take on jobs no one else wants or
will do. Institutional administrations are sometimes reluctant to
interfere with such individuals because they fear they will be
unable to find anyone else who will even attempt the job (Note
Case, 1975).

Because of the variety of institutional defenses, the Courts
have experimented with a variety of implementation and monitoring devices designed to provide facts for the court, or to act as
the court's eyes and ears in following implementation. Institutions
can be required to provide periodic progress reports. Ombuds-
men empowered to hear and investigate complaints can be appointed. The courts have the power to place institutions in
receivership. Someone can be appointed by the court to run the
institution. The variety of compliance devices and their formats
are reviewed in a Note (Note Case, 1975), and by Lottman (1976)
and Nathan (1979).

In the *Wyatt* case (Note Case, 1975), Judge Johnson appointed
Human Rights Committees who were to function as "standing
committees" at each of the institutions to review all research and
treatment programs. They were also to advise and assist inmates
who alleged that their legal rights had been violated or that the
Alabama Mental Health Board failed to comply with the judicially
ordered guidelines. While the responsibilities of this review committee were broad, its powers were not at all delineated. A note in
the *Yale Law Journal* (Note Case, 1975) examined the functioning

of these human rights committees with a particular emphasis on the one appointed for the Partlow State School and Hospital for the mentally retarded. The evaluation of the functioning of this group revealed the full range of problems in attempting to change a total institution.

Lottman (1976), who participated as an attorney in the *Wyatt* v *Stickney* case, and who was a member of the review panel appointed for the Willowbrook, New York, institution for the retarded, describes the more explicit powers granted that panel based on earlier experiences with the Wyatt case. He concludes:

> On paper, the Willowbrook court order seemed in April of 1975 to be a strong and specific statement of rights, and the Willowbrook Review Panel seemed to be a powerful and effective guarantor of those rights. The results, to date, however, have been less than satisfying, although the review panel mechanism still holds promise. It remains to be seen whether review panels are the answer to successful implementation in court decrees—in Willowbrook, in Nebraska, or elsewhere. (p.97)

Lottman's pessimism warns us to take a closer look at the problems which have emerged. Much of what follows will depend upon the Note Case (1975) evaluation of the *Wyatt* Human Rights Committee.

At first, Stonewall B. Stickney, Commissioner of the Alabama Board of Mental Health, was opposed to the court decision because he regarded it as an unwarranted intrusion of Federal power. However, since he was the defendant, he was under court orders to try to do something about Alabama institutions. Apparently, he came to see the court order as an opportunity, and he began fighting for increased budgets. It didn't take long for him and one of the state hospital superintendents, J. C. Folsom, to be fired by Governor Wallace, who, it seems, disagreed with the position Mr. Stickney took. Stickney was replaced by a Mr. Aderholt, who lasted about a year. Aderholt was replaced by Alabama National Guard General Hardin, a man politically close to Governor Wallace. General Hardin was available for the job since he had recently been forced to resign his post as State Finance Commissioner due to a conflict of interests (Note Case, 1975).

Lottman points out a key issue here, as did the Note Case. The courts can order mental health officials to comply, but if they don't have the funds there is not much the officials can do. A similar problem arose in the attempt to enforce the court order in *Welsch* v *Likins* (1974). There state officials were ordered to seek additional budgetary funds to improve the institutions. They sought the funds but were rejected by the governor and the state legislature. In the Willowbrook case in New York, Governor Rockefeller was named as a defendant and was directed to take all necessary steps to obtain sufficient funds, including making a submission for funds to the state legislature. What can the courts do if a state legislature refuses to supply the funds? It seems unlikely that a state legislature as a whole would be named defendants and ordered to produce a suitable budget, on pain of contempt. In Alabama, Governor Wallace supported the substantive goals of Judge Johnson's decree, although he stated his opposition to the intervention of the Federal Court. In fact, he gave $11 million in Federal revenue sharing funds to the Mental Health Board, and those funds were available for improvements (Note Case, 1975). It is apparent though that the issue of a constitutional right to treatment, and the problem of forcing sufficient funds to permit improvements through the courts, goes right to the heart of the balance of powers between the legislative, the executive, and the judiciary.

The relationship between the Human Rights Committee or the Review Panel and the institution it is meant to monitor presents a complex set of organizational as well as legal problems. In *Wyatt*, one Human Rights Committee consisted of a minister, a newspaper editor, three parents of retarded children (one of them resident in the institution), and a former resident of the institution. Initially they weren't paid, but later they received a per diem fee equal to that received by members of the Alabama Board of Mental Health. They also had no funds to hire staff at first, although they did have access to consultants. Their activities were thus considerably limited.

The Willowbrook panel consisted of two members appointed by defendants, three chosen by plaintiffs, and two recognized experts in the field of mental retardation, agreeable to both sides. Lottman points out that a seven-member citizens panel, even with authority to hire three full-time staff members, constitutes a slow moving, unresponsive body. It took them more than three months just to hire their first staff member.

Even after the panels began functioning, their powers were not carefully delineated, so it was not clear what they could do. The Alabama Human Rights Committees had no specific power to obtain any information, and they began by holding hearings. At first, staff cooperated with them, but as it became clear the Human Rights Committee and hospital authorities were adversaries, critical of the staff, their ability to obtain information was reduced. Hospital authorities resented their activities as encroachments on administrative prerogatives. Staff felt that the various decrees and the activities of the human rights committees were causing them to lose control. Staff, the institution's superintendent, and the committee began fighting covertly and overtly. Human rights committee members suspected that instances of abuse of residents increased, but they could get no evidence, since staff perceived them as the outside enemy, closed ranks, and refused to "inform" on each other.

The Willowbrook Review Panel was given access to all information and records, was permitted to visit any part of the institution at any time, was to be permitted to interview any resident or any institutional employee, and to conduct any other inquiries it deemed necessary. Neither panel could compel testimony, or take testimony under oath. Lottman doesn't report that the staff resisted, but he does complain that cooperation from the Department of Mental Hygiene was less than complete.

Both the Human Rights Committees and the Review Panel were charged with reviewing and evaluating progress in implementing the Court's decree. Institutional authorities were also charged with filing periodic progress reports. Both the Human Rights Committee and the Panel were empowered to review and comment on the progress reports and to make their own recommendations. In both settings several problems emerged. First, the review bodies and the institutions would disagree on the status of implementation of proposals. Specifics concerning number of personnel or other physical conditions (e.g., number of toilets) could be determined. However, how can one determine whether a humane and caring environment has been established? In many instances, the review bodies and the administration simply disagreed, and there was no way to settle their disagreements without resorting to further litigation, or to additional, expensive evaluation.

Second, the review bodies were unclear whether they were to emphasize the best available approach consistent with the intent of the court, or whether they were to approve minimally acceptable methods. In the Willowbrook situation, panel members were uncertain about trying to influence Mental Hygiene decisions in advance, or allowing the Mental Hygiene Department to follow through on its own ideas, and then to object later, if they disagreed.

In the Alabama situation some very curious and complex problems of a related kind arose. Judge Johnson's order was based upon the recommendations of a variety of experts. These experts were concerned both about in-hospital care and about moving toward deinstitutionalization. In some instances, the Human Rights Committee felt that Alabama authorities complied by "dumping" patients in inadequate community facilities. They even suspected hospital authorities of arranging it so that disturbed patients would be sent unsupervised into local communities in order to stimulate resistance to change. However, they were uncertain about their authority to follow patients into the community. Moreover, if the constitutional requirement was treatment in the least restricted facility, which had precedence—institutional improvement, or the provision of community based care? And who would decide whether a given modification led to one goal or to the other?

The Alabama plan also gave rise to a peculiar problem of another kind. The order required that treatment plans be made for each patient. It also required that personnel be hired according to a predetermined table of organization, and with specified qualifications. Personnel were hired and some progress was made in designing individual treatment programs. However, it quickly became apparent that the personnel suitable for doing patient evaluation and designing the treatment programs were not necessarily trained to carry out the treatment programs. One could not determine in advance what sort of treatment programs were necessary, but having hired the personnel it was not clear the treatment programs could be carried out by those personnel. The order presented a logical bind.

The standards for personnel were based on recommendations of the major professional organizations, each of whom had their own interests in promoting professional standards in training and qualifications. The political interests of the professional organizations were not obvious from their testimony as experts. Graduation from most accredited training programs in clinical psychology, or in psychiatric social work, or the completion of a residency in psychiatry in most training institutions which emphasize psychotherapy with highly verbal patients will do little to provide the training necessary to work with chronic mental patients or with the institutionalized retarded. The court accepted the words of "foremost authorities on mental health in the United States," as Judge Johnson characterized the witnesses who testified at the hearing he held. The Court could not have been aware of the experts' tendencies to promote professional self interests.

The Human Rights Committees did have access to some resources which were helpful. The Court had appointed the U.S. District Attorney counsel for the committee. In one instance, they were able to call on the FBI to help them in an investigation of charges relating to patient deaths. The Committee also had direct access to the Court. The Mental Health Association helped to provide consultants to the Committee. The Committee had a distant relationship with the attorneys for the plaintiffs because the court wished to keep the Committee as the court's agent, and not the plaintiffs'. The Committee couldn't really use the plaintiffs' attorneys' resources very well because the Committee didn't have its own priorities worked out. There was thus a complex relationship between parties on all sides, which resulted in uncertainty and in delays, if not in inaction. Apparently the presence of a newspaperman on the committee proved one of the group's strongest assets, since he could reach the general public by way of regular stories detailing the institution's problems (Note Case, 1975).

Some change was accomplished in the first few years. More staff were hired and institutional conditions improved. Sanitation, living quarters, food, and general decency in staff attitudes toward patients seems to have improved. Overcrowding and overwork was reduced by discharging some patients. Treatment plans were made but implementation was slow. The Human Rights Committee said that much of the treatment was of a token nature, and indeed this issue provoked further conflict later on.

The events in Alabama institutions took place during the time the District Court's ruling was under appeal. Not sure whether the Circuit Court would uphold him, Judge Johnson may have been somewhat more restrained in enforcing his order than he might have been in a less novel legal situation. The Circuit Court upheld his decision (*Wyatt* v *Aderholt*, 1974), but progress continued to be slow.

In November 1978, Judge Johnson presided over a hearing to assess compliance with his April 1972 order. The hearing caused bitter controversy amongst groups of expert witnesses testifying on both sides (e.g., Ellis, 1979; Roos, 1979). The plaintiff's attorneys had gone to great lengths to sponsor studies showing the nature of treatment and its inadequacies, while defense witnesses claimed the nature of patient problems was such that the treatment efforts were useless and would be bound to fail. The defendant's experts felt that a program of enrichment within the institution was the best that could be offered; they suggested an adequate set of conditions meeting the requirement of the least restrictive environment for the chronic patients remaining in the institution. The defendant's experts did not feel community based treatment was either necessary or desirable for all patients.

Following the hearing, and apparently after long deliberation, Judge Johnson said:

> Based on all the evidence presented in this case, the Court makes the following findings of fact and conclusions of law. The hazardous and deplorable conditions which existed at Partlow in 1972 have to some degree been ameliorated. The severe overcrowding has been eliminated. At the same time the size of the staff has increased although there are still shortages of trained personnel in some fields [especially physical and recreational therapists]. Concomitantly, the physical conditions have improved. However the evidence reflects continued serious areas of non-compliance. (*Wyatt* v *Ireland, II*, 1975, p.5 Memorandum Opinion)

His order continued:

> The Court now finds and concludes that defendants are in substantial and serious noncompliance with the orders entered in this

case over seven years ago, in several critical areas. Among these are:

1. Failure to provide adequate habilitation programming;
2. Insufficiently trained staff;
3. Failure to move residents from the larger institutions to less restrictive settings;
4. Failure to provide privacy for residents;
5. Inadequate policies and practices concerning the administration of medication—this includes serious overmedication;
6. Failure to adequately protect residents from abuse by staff members;
7. Failure to provide an adequate dental care program;
8. Failure to provide adequate medical supervision and care.

(Wyatt v Ireland, II, p. 14)

As part of his order, Judge Johnson appointed a special master (in this case, Governor James of Alabama) to oversee compliance with the order issued originally over seven and one half years earlier. (The Governor was appointed special master about a year before this book was written. According to plaintiff's attorneys, Governor James had as yet not given the problem his full attention.)

Advantages and limits of judicial remedies. When constitutional or statutory deficiencies have been found in the operation of human service institutions, courts have resorted to the use of monitors, special masters, and receivers to aid in formulating enforcing or even administering remedies (Nathan, 1979). These special officers serve as extensions of the courts, and judges have a great deal of discretion in specifying their duties and their powers. In general, powers and duties are assigned judiciously and in proportion to the complexity of meeting judicial orders, and the history of recalcitrance in complying. Judges, respecting the separation of powers, and well aware the judiciary cannot undertake to administer institutions, are reluctant to intrude unnecessarily into administrative prerogatives even when they seek to remedy constitutional or statutory deficiencies.

Because courts are reluctant to intrude unnecessarily, they have limited the powers assigned to monitors or masters to those deemed minimally necessary to achieve compliance with orders. Some monitors or masters may be limited to an information gathering function, but with power to gain access to all necessary information. Because a master or a monitoring committee is an arm of the court, it has direct access to the judge. Moreover, any of its formal findings of fact, and its judgments about the degree of compliance, have great weight in influencing subsequent court actions. Their very presence may motivate efforts to comply.

A special master has additional functions beyond fact finding. The special master can negotiate, oversee, mediate, or arbitrate plans for compliance, and can exercise great influence on the nature of those plans. In some instances, masters have been empowered to recommend to the court the removal or transfer of any staff member or employee as necessary to obtain implementation of the judge's orders.

A court-appointed receiver assumes all the duties and powers of the official he displaces. The receiver has full administrative power, and in addition can call on the court for further assistance in obtaining the powers and the resources necessary to implement the court's order. Judge Johnson, for example, threatened to sell lands belonging to the state hospital to obtain funds necessary to bring the institution to minimally adequate standards.

Nathan (1979) believes that masters have been effective in achieving institutional reforms, but his conclusions are at variance with those of other observers (e.g., Note Case, 1975; Lottman, 1976; Note, 1977) who are considerably less sanguine about the results in mental hospitals and state schools for the retarded. The monitoring instrument is undoubtedly a powerful one, but as yet we have no systematic information about the best composition of the group, the qualifications of its leader, the powers and duties best assigned for what purposes, and its best organizational location. It is conceivable that monitoring can be effective in limiting abuses and in overseeing the installation of readily observable changes (e.g., the number of toilets or reduction in patient staff ratios). The formulation of plans for remedies may be accomplished with the use of expert consultants. But the understanding of organizational and bureaucratic dynamics requires another order of knowledge.

The implementation of plans with a spirit that will be in keeping with the form may require inspired line clinical leadership and a sufficient number of dedicated lieutenants to supervise day-by-day activity (Levine, 1980). The combination of inspired clinical leadership with ready access to judicial power has impressive potential for achieving change even in the most highly resistant institutions. Nathan's excellent review touches on complex legal, ethical, and practical problems in using the instrument. There is probably enough experience now so that a theoretical framework for the use of monitors and masters could be developed. The ideal master may be an individual with legal training, administrative background, and substantive clinical and leadership skills and knowledge. In a few years, clinical psychologist-lawyers emerging out of J.D.-Ph.D. programs may be ideally suited. It is clear that the role of change agent requires a new professional who truly integrates several disciplines in his or her training and who brings to bear a wholistic perspective on the problem of change.

SOME FINAL COMMENTS

Roscoe Pound (1910) formulated the distinction between the law on the books and the law in action. Legal rules can serve justice only within the operational context of a social organization. The best of rules can be subverted in their application. The chapters above have described instances in mental health when good intentions went awry, and instances in the law when ideals accomplished nothing. The issues we have been examining in chapters 5 and 6 fall in the common area between the law and mental health systems. There are many reasons for the failures in implementation, but an important one is that each system—each societal institution, the mental health service system, and the law as a social institution—is designed "to do its own thing." Each has been asked to do something foreign to itself in the intersecting area, with the result that the foreign element is not as well integrated into the system as it needs to be for full effectiveness.

The purpose of the court is to see that justice is done. It fulfills the purpose by trying to preserve equities in relationships, and by trying to see to it that we live by the rule of law, that we are all afforded equal protection under the law, and that we are not subject to caprice and arbitrary action, especially by the state. In the field of mental health, the courts acted under the state's police power to protect society, and under the parens patriae power, the state's obligation as the ultimate parent to care for its citizens. The courts clearly had a role in the commitment process, in seeing to it that individual rights were protected and that the state fulfilled its obligations.

The problem is not with the concept. The problem is with the implementation of the concept through the legal system as a social organization. The legal system is the home of members of the legal profession. It is the institution within which members of the legal profession earn their livings, and it is within that social organization that the culture of the legal profession exerts its influence on the behavior, the attitudes, and the very thought processes of its members.

For most lawyers and judges, mental health law does not stand very high in the scale of values, interest, or prestige within the profession. Judges are required to decide whether to commit or not, whether to release or not, and in recent years to determine the most suitable treatment for patients. None of these are tasks for which judges and lawyers receive great rewards, nor are they tasks for which most have any training or special education. I do not have any data to support me, but I imagine that the routine work of commitment hearings and the like is a bore. It is unlikely that judges will be rewarded with a higher bench because they do good work in routine commitment or habeas corpus hearings. Few lawyers will make a career of representing relatively difficult, indigent clients and expect to earn a partnership in a prestigious law firm. Within the culture of the law, there is not much in it for lawyers and judges. It is understandable that such chores are given low priority in the allocation of legal energy. The result shows in the perfunctory way the duty of safeguarding legal rights is carried out.

The legal profession also has its own discipline and its own aims. The adversarial model's aim is to present the best case for each side of a question on the assumption that the truth will emerge from hard, fair, even mental combat. Operationally, however, lawyers want to win. It is not clear what it means to win for a client unless it is to obtain a disposition meeting the client's needs. To win in court, but not to have an alternative for the client, may be legitimate within the norms of the legal profession, but in this intersecting area, the concept of winning needs to be rethought. Lawyers may well have won paper victories for clients, a result which enhances the lawyer's status within the profession, but doesn't obviously serve the client.

When lawyers and judges undertook to reform institutions, they did it with assumptions and tools fashioned for other purposes. It is one thing to give over control of a complicated estate to a court appointed official for administration, or even to take over a railroad for purposes of getting a grip on its finances. It is quite another to order intangibles such as modern therapy delivered with skill and good will. It is one thing to threaten a corporate official with some penalty. It is quite another to threaten a cabinet secretary, a governor, or a legislator. It is certainly the province of the judiciary to say what the law is and what is required, but we live in a system of separation of powers and each component has its own powers. Officials in other branches exercise considerable autonomy. In any event, courts are not generally equipped to exercise long-term supervision over other agencies of government, although they appear to be learning how to do it in school desegregation cases. Perhaps the courts will learn how to supervise change in mental hospitals and schools for the retarded as well. For now, the modes of thinking, the theories of change, and the instruments have not been fully effective. However, at the same time we point to limitations, we must also acknowledge that litigation has resulted in improvements in the physical condition of institutions and patients, and that is no mean achievement.

It is necessary to ask whether or not it makes sense to hope for reform by putting more and more responsibility onto legal process, as in more stringent due process requirements for commitments, and in asking courts to say what good treatment is. An *amicus curiae* brief in *Bartley* v *Kremens* (1975) argued that one could not rely on mental health professionals to make decisions to institutionalize children simply on their parents' request because mental health professionals follow institution policies, yield to parental pressure, or make decisions based on the inability to command alternative resources. The brief asserted the court would have superior power to hear arguments, to determine whether care could be provided outside an institution, to ascertain the care available in the institution, to assess the home, and the child's and parent's feelings for each other. The brief described the hearing mechanism as a forum to understand the family situation, and to explore alternatives. The brief characterized the hearing officer as someone who would have the power to order the exploration of alternative resources, who could pressure public agencies stalled in bureaucratic delays, or who could even mandate the creation of the necessary resources (Wald & Friedman, 1976).

The courts may have the power and the flexibility to act to make things better, but there is nothing in our experience to suggest that the courts as they stand are the best agencies to treat social problems. The Juvenile Court, designed as a therapeutic agency, never bore out the hopes of its founders, except in a few isolated cases (Levine & Levine, 1970). The family courts, faced daily with the problem of making dispositions for thousands of youth never used whatever powers they might have had to order the creation of services, or even to supervise the institutions to which they committed youth (Polier, 1964). The juvenile and family courts were designed to serve rather than to punish, and these courts handled nothing but juvenile and family problems. We have no reason to believe that ordinary courts, busy with a variety of other matters, would devote time and attention to the complex tasks of seeing to it that the best alternatives would be found for each case. It may be that we need a different institution which is neither court nor clinic, but is some true amalgam of the two, and which is operated by individuals involved in the best of the law and the best of the mental health fields.

Beyond the rhetoric of a brief, we may note that the legal profession is very protective of its own interests and is not any more given to reform of itself than any other profession. The difference, of course, is that no other profession has as ready access to the coercive powers of the state. First-year law school textbooks on torts have many cases on medical malpractice, but none on legal malpractice. The coercive powers that might be used to control abuse in a field will not be readily employed to reform the legal profession.

The brief written for Donaldson for his Supreme Court case (Ennis et al., 1975) cites a 1961 Florida State Bar Association report critical of Florida state institutions. The brief discusses provisions of then recently revised Florida state laws that provided for liability for mental health professionals who did not act in good-faith compliance with the treatment provisions of the revised act. The Florida Bar Association was not equally indignant about the perfunctory nature of court hearings and the perfunctory participation of Florida attorneys and judges in such hearings (Miller, 1976). The legal profession can be criticized for being self-protective and self-serving by focusing exclusive attention on the deficiencies of mental health professionals without taking an equally hard look at the deficiencies within the legal institution. What is sauce for the goose is sauce for the gander. If coercive legal action is useful in reforming the field of mental health, shouldn't it be equally useful in reforming the field of law, also an element in the context in which mental health services are delivered?

The mental health professions exist to heal, to relieve suffering, to help others toward greater personal fulfillment, and to care for those in need unable to care for themselves. The society at large has delegated these very parental functions to the profession. However, the mental health professions also exercise a great deal of social control. The institutional system serves the function of removing and holding the deviant and the repulsive. The publically supported mental health service system serves as an arm to implement the police powers of the state. Most of the important legal decisions leading to reform have depended upon the protection of patient rights when the state incarcerates through the mental hospital or the state school system. The U.S. Supreme Court pointedly refused to recognize a right to treatment in *O'Connor* v *Donaldson* (1975), but it based its decision on the lack of right of the state to incarcerate without sufficient reason. It is the responsibility for controlling people that has gotten the mental health system and the profession into difficulty.

Just as with the legal profession, so the mental health professions also live out their culture through social institutions. The mental health professions place important value on the healing function, and much less on the custodial function. The existence of chronic, intractable problems among their patients is an embarassment to the field and a blow to its prestige. Moreover, those with the more chronic problems tend to be the poor, the powerless, and those with generally low if not degraded social status. The low status of the patient population rubs off on the caretakers. In general, the state hospitals and the state schools for the retarded are not prestigious places to work. Those employed in public institutions tend to be considered less able than those working in private sector agencies, or in private practice. Just as there is not much in it for lawyers to go into the mental health legal field, there is not much in it for a mental health professional to go into a public system that tends to be the repository for the unwanted.

Just as lawyers want to win, so do mental health professionals wish to cure. The profession is socialized into an acute treatment model. Much training goes on with good cases, meaning cases that enable the budding professional to exercise the skills the profession values the highest. There is not much professional satisfaction in taking care of a patient population that is relatively unresponsive to the most valued forms of treatment. It is discouraging to use tools which are ineffective. Burn-out is a prominent problem among those who work with chronic patient populations. The results of treatment far too often fall short of the ideal. It is easy enough for the professional to busy him or herself with whatever can be done, and to ignore the daily conditions of life, abdicating responsibility for basic care to lesser-trained and lesser-paid persons. It is easy to accept that that's the best that can be done, and to let it go at that.

Mental health professionals, with rare exception, are not social reformers, nor do modern day mental health professionals see it as their duty to fight against poor conditions, or to blow the whistle.[4] In many institutions, there is a live-and-let-live attitude. Professionals, if not covering up for each other, are reluctant to be critical of others. Many recognize that resources are lacking, or use that as a rationalization to excuse colleagues or subordinates

---

4. The Mental Health Systems Act (1980) contains a provision protecting the employment of whistleblowers (§ 307 (b)(5)).

whose performance is inadequate, or even outrageous. Blatt (1970) has pointed to the many ways in which institutional practice can lead to the dehumanization of the other and to callousness toward conditions that are shocking to outsiders. The conditions of providing care are accepted; it is a rare administrator who accepts the responsibility for correcting poor conditions, or for rousing public and political support for institutional reform. Occasionally some do so successfully, but their efforts are not usually welcomed by bureaucratic and political superiors more concerned that something got in the papers than about the condition that attracted newspaper attention in the first place. It is not scandalous conditions that are troublesome, it is scandal.

Because legislators in some states do not give their institutions high priority for funds, and because professional mental health workers are not prone to leading political battles for improved conditions, it is essential that the profession does have an outside guardian overlooking its efforts. It is not a bad thing to have someone who does not share the profession's assumptions and culture to look in and say, "Those are unconscionable conditions that must change." In that sense, litigation has served an extraordinarily useful function, since self-policing and self-correction have failed. The difficulty is that mandated changes from outside tend to be resisted, and may not have enduring value for practice. While some have felt comfortable working with lawyers to achieve change, many see the changes lawyers desire as unrealistic and unnecessary.

Lawyers and judges may demand change, but it is line mental health workers who have to implement the changes. If they do not believe in them, or see the changes as impossible because there is no inspiring clinical leadership to show how the new is to be implemented, or if they see their jobs threatened, as when an order to place patients in a community results in a reduced hospital census and the threat of closing their institution, then change is resisted. The order itself is not enough to win the hearts and minds of those who must implement it. We have not yet learned how to mandate attitudes and feelings.

Sarason (1978) has suggested that it is inappropriate to apply the technology of problem solution to problems in the social realm, especially when the social problems will never go away.

Note that we are faced with a sleight of hand in which 60 percent of mental patients disappear from mental hospitals. The magician points to their disappearance and distracts our attention from the bulge in nursing home populations and psychiatric ghettos. Litigation has contributed its share to the motivation of states to release patients into the community. Legislation has also provided state-level mental health administrators with powerful fiscal incentives to release patients into the community. In one relationship, the legal and mental health systems have been adversaries, but in another, the two systems have worked hand in hand. It is important to appreciate latent as well as manifest aspects of a relationship.

The best of ideas, and the best of intentions, may be, if not smashed, then often damaged on the hard rocks of complex social reality. Our methods, focused as they are on the narrow considerations dictated by our disciplines, give us limited perspectives and limited answers. Our scientific orientation presumes that all we think we know today has superceded the faulty knowledge of the past. The history of similar solutions having been tried, having failed, and having been replaced is forgotten or ignored. We have yet to learn that opting for the same solutions without doing something different will result in the same consequences. It is not that we can ever anticipate error-free actions. Not at all. The problems are so complex and the variables so many that interactions cannot be predicted. We should, however, begin to anticipate the worst of our errors. Whether we have or not may become clear as we examine the recommendations of the President's Commission on Mental Health, the most recent authoritative body to review the field of mental health.

Chapter 7

REPORT
OF THE PRESIDENT'S COMMISSION
ON MENTAL HEALTH
The Development of Public Policy

The President's Commission on Mental Health was established by
President Jimmy Carter by Executive Order No. 11973 in February 1977, a few months after he assumed office. The creation of
the Commission so early in his tenure and the appointment of the
First Lady to be its honorary Chairperson reflected the commitment of the Carters, both of whom had been active in mental
health affairs in Georgia. The President's Commission Report
(1978a) was submitted in April 1978 and it was soon on its way to
influencing prospective legislation. Immediately after its appearance, the Secretary of what was then Health, Education and
Welfare (now Health and Human Services) established an Interagency Task Force to analyze the implications for HEW programs
of the report's recommendations, and to propose legislation that
would be responsive to the Commission's recommendations and
intent. The Task Force was chaired by Gerald Klerman, Administrator of the Alcohol, Drug Abuse and Mental Health Administration; it included representatives of the major divisions within
HEW: Health, Education, Human Development, Legislation,
Management and Budget, Planning and Evaluation, Social Security
Administration, and Health Care Financing Administration (HEW
Task Force, 1979).

This chapter relies heavily on a paper by the same title by M. Levine and
collaborators, to be published in *Health Policy Quarterly* in 1981.

Subsequently, Mrs. Carter testified for newly submitted legislation before Senator Kennedy's Subcommittee on Health and Scientific Research, with news photos showing the four volumes of the President's Commission Report in front of her as she gave her testimony. She was reportedly unfazed when Senator Kennedy inquired about her feelings that the President's budget requested an increase for mental health programs, in contrast to the austerity budgets recommended for many other social programs (U.S. Senate Committee on Labor and Human Resources, 1980). Her testimony was an event in itself. It was the first time a First Lady had testified before Congress in support of a major piece of legislation. The new Mental Health Systems Act, recently passed by Congress, very clearly shows the marks of its recommendations. The President's Commission Report did not recommend any radical departure from existing mental health programs. Rather it reviewed and endorsed the variety of reforms that have been apparent in mental health since the 1960s.

The President's Commission Report, and its preparation, deserves the closest analysis precisely because it appears to be having an important effect at a national level. Although the future of mental health funding is uncertain at this writing (just after the 1980 election), the Report pretty much follows federal policy developed by the professional leadership that dominated the first twenty-five years of NIMH (Foley, 1975). This influence persists, just as the influence of the President's Commission is likely to persist, if for no other reason than that the summary of this prestigious group's findings now appear in the congressional committee reports constituting the legislative history.

In this chapter, we are less interested in examining the specific legislative recommendations that eventually emerged than in trying to understand the process of mental health planning within the political context in which mental health funds are allocated. As we will see, the Commission was not only constrained by the practicalities of what already exists, and the necessity to develop realistic and palatable recommendations, but it also was constrained by the rationale behind its formation, and by its methods of working. I will concentrate on the last two features.

The federal budget for Alcohol, Drug Abuse and Mental Health (ADAMHA) is now over a billion dollars a year, with approximately half of that going for mental health services. The federal budget is very large, and there is no reason to believe that such a very large budget will not be subject to all of the special interest pressures shaping other large federal budgets. Mental health planning is not a straightforward venture carried forth by disinterested, public-spirited citizens and professionals. The "Nation's foremost mental health authorities and other volunteers interested in mental health" (President's Commission Report) may be exactly that, but they are also making decisions about the allocation of large sums of money, and few are disinterested under those circumstances. The deficiencies in the data base, in the documentation, and in the analysis of data in most of the Task Panel Reports may be taken as the hallmarks of a political process, only partly guided by professional standards of excellence.

The composition of the Commission. The Commission was composed by a small ad hoc committee chaired by Dr. John Gardner, a psychologist, who was then Chairman of Common Cause, a citizen's political-action group. Dr. Gardner had served as Secretary of HEW in the past. The screening committee submitted a small pool winnowed from 1000 names to the President and to Mrs. Carter for final selection. The twenty-member Commission included eight women and twelve men. In contrast to the Joint Commission on Mental Health and Illness, whose places were reserved specifically for representatives of various professional organizations (e.g. American Medical Association, American Psychiatric Association, American Psychological Association, National League for Nursing etc.), the President's Commission was selected to achieve, in addition to their knowledgeability of the mental health field, a balance in representation for sex, race, and ethnic and professional background. The President's Commissioners, in contrast to members of the Joint Commission, were *not* representatives of professional organizations.

The Committee's three psychiatrists, all well-qualified by virtue of training, experience, and professional prominence, included a director of a community mental health center who had been a past president of the National Council of Community Mental Health Centers (Allen Biegel); a state commissioner of mental health who was a black woman (Mildred Mitchell-Bateman); and a representative of academic medicine, who had also served on the Joint Commission, and is widely acknowledged to be both influential and knowledgeable about mental health politics on a national level (George Tarjan).

The Commission included consumer representatives in the person of Priscilla Allen, a former patient now active in lobbying for mental health programs in California, and recognized for her views on consumer participation and advocacy in mental health; and Thomas Conlan, a member of Alcoholics Anonymous, a lawyer, a member of the Ohio Board of Regents, and a bank director. As a leading citizen-volunteer, he has served on many committees on subjects related to education, health, alcoholism, and mental health.

Other citizen volunteers included individuals who can be characterized objectively as members of a mental health power structure (Graziano, 1969). Virginia Dayton is on at least one mental health agency board, on a statewide mental health advisory council, and on the Board of Directors of United Way. LaDonna Harris, a member of many boards, wife of a U.S. Senator, and a recognized crusader for human rights, is also an active member of the Comanche tribe. Beverly Long, a Georgian who worked with the Carters on the development of mental health programs in Georgia, is a former president of the state mental health association, and served as president of the National Mental Health Association. Florence Mahoney, now in her 70s, has been an advocate for the aging and has been co-chairperson of the National Committee Against Mental Illness (an organization similar to the National Mental Health Association) since 1950. Another lay person is Glenn Watts, a union president, a member of the executive council of the AFL-CIO, and Chairman of the Executive Committee of the United Way of America. Jose Cabranes serves on the boards of a settlement house and a community hospital, and is legal adviser and Director of Government Relations at Yale. Reymundo Rodriguez is associated with the Hogg Foundation for Mental Health and is also active in statewide and regional planning for human services.

The various professions were also well represented by prominent individuals: John Conger (a psychologist), Martha Mitchell (a nurse), Harold Richman (a social worker), Ruth Love (a former superintendent of schools associated with programs for disadvantaged and minority youth), Franklin E. Vilas (an Episcopal minister active in pastoral counseling programs), and Charles V. Wille (a sociologist, Professor of Education and Urban Studies at Harvard, and active in mental health, minority mental health programs, and in the development of black colleges). Julius Richmond, Professor of Psychiatry at Harvard Medical School, who became Surgeon General of the United States, served ex-officio on the Commission.

The Commission's Executive Director was Thomas E. Bryant, M.D., J.D., who had been active in health, mental health, mental retardation, and drug abuse. A graduate of Emory University in Atlanta, Georgia, he had many ties to government and to professional associations. He was a confidante and adviser to the Carters on mental health before his appointment to the President's Commission.

The presence of women, blacks, hispanics, and an Amerindian on the Commission now reflects a new-found consciousness of minority interests. While there may have been some members of these groups on committees and working groups appointed by the Joint Commission, they were not appointed because of their minority status, and the concerns of minority groups, nascent in the late 1950s, did not influence the work of the Joint Commission. A recognition of the concerns and interests of our diverse population, however, is now both morally and politically necessary. The comparison should also alert us to the variety of interests reflected in mental health policymaking today as compared to the past.

The Commission was assisted in its work by 35 Task Panels, appointed to develop recommendations in their specific areas. Many of the panelists were prominent contributors to the scientific and professional literature. However, lay persons, activists in various causes, administrators, journalists, and representatives of a great many organizations and associations participated. The support staff for the President's Commission and the Task Panels was provided by the Secretary of HEW. The Task Panel reports (President's Commission, 1978b) were intended to provide the data base for the Commission, although its members were also expected to bring their own supply of first-hand experience to the problem.

Methods of working. In understanding the President's Commission Report, it is instructive to examine how the Commission worked, and how the report related to the data and the recommendations provided by the Task Panel reports. In contrast to the six-year life of the Joint Commission, the President's Commission made its full report within fourteen months of its creation. The President's Commission was under some pressure to report early. In fact, it issued an early report to influence the fiscal 1979 budget, and it developed an interim report earlier for similar purposes. Its relatively tight schedule and its need to report early might have influenced some of the way it worked. The quality of its work may well have been enhanced, as we shall note, by a more leisurely schedule, but in the political world, in which the budget ax threatens to fall momentarily, leisurely contemplation is considered an unaffordable luxury.

The Commission and the Task Panels worked simultaneously. The Commission held regional hearings as a forum for testimony from professionals, consumers, family members, and political figures. The Commission also had the benefit of some special studies from the National Academy of Sciences, acknowledged in the Report, but never published as part of the Appendices. Each Task Panel met twice, usually for two- to three-day work sessions. Members contributed position papers. After a discussion, a panel member, usually the chairperson, but sometimes a Commission liaison staff person, took responsibility for drafting a report. Mrs. Carter and other members of the Commission participated in the deliberations of at least some of the Task Panels. Actually, the final panel reports were not prepared in time for the Commission to work from the written documents. The chairpersons of the Task Panels presented their findings and recommendations orally. Despite the fact that the final written reports were not available, one can trace the recommendations of many of the expert Task Panels in the Commission's final report. From the viewpoint of the Task Panelists, "success" was measured by how much influence they had on the Commission to adopt certain principles or recommendations. As we have noted, the majority of the Commissioners were not professionals who would be especially sensitive to data based arguments. It was never clear exactly what would influence the Commissioners, but panelists were aware the Commission would balance varied demands, and would take into account various political considerations in their final recommendations. One of the minority group Task Panels complained that it felt its views did not receive fuller consideration because that minority group was not represented on the Commission itself (Vol. III, p.777). Its complaint reflected the view that political considerations were critical, and that it was within the rules of the game to express such considerations in print.

The Task Panel Reports. The quality of the Task Panel reports vary widely; apparently its members understood their instructions very differently. The reports range from very brief ones, which look as if they had been written by someone on the plane on the way to the meeting, to well-thought out analytic reviews. Some consist of little more than a list of recommendations. No more than a third of the Task Panel reports would pass muster as scholarly documents. The preparation of the reports was sloppy. Many are poorly written. Citations made in the body of the report do not appear in the bibliographies. Citations for key points are often to unpublished sources. To be fair, it must be stated that some of the Task Panels did not expect their reports to be published.

Few of the Task Panel reports offer a careful, thorough, critical review of the existing literature, an analysis of the issues, or a thoughtful weighing of alternatives. Many are advocacy documents that assert much, are couched in rhetoric, and purport to cite data, often in uncritical fashion and with little regard for the limits of inference from the data cited.

It is not that one cannot learn from the Task Panel reports. The report on the Scope of the Problem (Vol. II) contains a great deal of very useful data on the significance of the distribution of age in the population for future needs for service. The special study of alternative services presents a great deal of interesting descriptive material. Much of it was gathered from those who offer the alternative services, and much of it was presented from that viewpoint as well. The report on Families, Children and Adolescents (Vol. III) may have many intelligent recommendations, but it is all but useless as a source document, despite the fact that the panel included a large number of distinguished scholars. The Task Panel report on Learning Failure seemed painfully amateurish (Vol. III). The reports on special populations (Vol. III)— Women, Asian/Pacific Americans, Black Americans, Americans of Euro-ethnic Origin, Hispanic Americans, American Indians and Alaskan Natives, and the Physically Handicapped—varied in their quality.

The Task Panel on Women presented a well-reasoned position, but one that was dominated by feminist rhetoric. Alternative positions were neither presented nor criticized, nor was there any exploration of the limits of the feminist position, or the problems it created as well as solved. Its political character is well illustrated by the inclusion of the entire list of resolutions adopted by the 1977 Houston National Women's Conference as an appendix to its report.

The Euro-ethnic report was perfunctory, perhaps reflecting the lack of political organization of these groups for mental health services. The reports on the other minority groups sometimes contained some useful data, and some interesting observations on the cultures of different groups. There were some insightful specifications of the issues in developing culturally appropriate services. Too often, however, the task panelists, composed entirely or nearly so of members of the ethnic or racial group, indulged their prejudices, with little attempt at scholarly analysis of the existing data base or the limitations of the positions that were shrilly advocated.

The Task Panel report on the elderly provided a bare minimum of useful information or analysis (Vol. III). The Task Panel on Access and Barriers to Care provided an overly simplistic discussion of stigma, one which did not deal with the many intriguing problems in the literature.

The report on Migrant and Seasonal Workers (Vol. III) contained careful description and analysis of the problems of this group, and of cultural and economic patterns that influenced the nature of mental health problems and the receptivity of given subpopulations to services. This group was similar to the Women's panel, outspoken in its assertion that the argicultural labor system would require considerable reform before mental health services could make any dent in mental health problems. The panel on Legal and Ethical issues also presented a reasoned and forceful case for continued efforts on the legal front, but it did not deal with any of the criticisms of the results of litigation. The report of the Task Panel on Prevention was one of the more cohesive and creative essays on the problems and prospects for prevention. But it too stopped short of critically reviewing the basic data in the field. (See Levine & Perkins, 1980 for a review and critique of the Task Panel Report.)

The inadequacies of the Task Panel reports are understandable, given the limited amount of time they had to work. It is surprising that some are as well done and as useful as they are. However, other conditions may also have contributed to the character of the reports. First, almost all of the Task Panel reports can be characterized as advocacy rather than review documents. Each one concludes that there are inadequate numbers of workers in that field and inadequate resources devoted to it, considering its central importance. The legal panel asked for more lawyers and the public relations panel (Vol. IV) for more public relations people, as did just about every other speciality and interest group. There was no statement that a particular direction would be likely to result in a dead end, or that it had distinct limits that militated against its further development. There were no recommendations against, only urgent recommendations for more. If there was a villain, it was the private practitioner, interested in serving middle-class clients, one-on-one, and on a (high) fee-for-service basis. Otherwise, the panelists seemed to be working with the hallowed principle, "Never knock another guy's hustle, and certainly not your own."

Second, there was little critical analysis of the data bases in different fields, except perhaps to indicate that we don't know enough about most things and that more research funds were necessary. There are many excellent suggestions for research, for service, and for policy analysis scattered throughout the reports, but these are rarely well developed in context, and do not often derive from a careful and critical analysis of a body of literature.

The Task Panelists, as a general rule, did not seem to see it as

their function to state the limits of knowledge underlying particular recommendations, or to explore alternatives, or even to
consider possible unintended consequences. Recommendations
for the development of natural community support systems, the
Commission's first major recommendation, ignore the adequacy
of such systems to deal with certain problems such as chronic
illness. The assumption that neighbors will want to help each
other ignores much of what we know about how communities are
fragmented, with different segments fighting each other. Further,
the problems for which community action and natural support
are useful, and problems for which they have not been useful, or
have not been studied, were not differentiated. People turn to
public services when their own resources are inadequate to meet
the demands made of them. Perhaps it is too much to ask for a
detailed analysis of the issues, but the Commission's first recommendation was for action to enhance support systems. Was that
recommendation based on a careful consideration of what we
think we know and what we don't know, or was it just based on
the faddishness of the concept?

The Task Panel on Prevention, which wrote one of the more
coherent reports, failed to mention that no prevention study in
psychology or in the other social sciences had yet to demonstrate
any long-range effect of preventive programs. Moreover, their
thinking failed to take into account the problem of the specificity
of environmental and personal interventions, demonstrated in so
many other fields. There are good arguments to be made against
the possibility that prevention of emotional problems in childhood would have discernible effects in adulthood. For example,
although boys far outnumber girls in rates of teacher-judged
maladjustment in school, in adult life, women make use of mental
health services in as great or greater number than do men. A good
adjustment in childhood doesn't necessarily presage a good adjustment in adult life. In its concern to see that the concept of
prevention was protected against the legion of its enemies, the
Task Panel may have overpromised and so hurt its cause (Levine &
Perkins, 1980).

Several of the Task Panels called for more community control
over service delivery, ignoring the problems of establishing workable community control. There is no consideration of the well-

known abuses and limitations of community control, including the fact that participants are not representative of their communities, that the distinction between policy and operational roles is sometimes lost, and that community board members have on occasion intervened in the hiring process, making patronage possible and interfering with line discipline. These problems must be identified and analyzed before they can be avoided by current planners. This is what the Task Panels should have done and did not.

There were also other areas where the Task Panels failed. The points of view expressed in many of the reports on research were based on the research of some of the panel members. While those panel members were undoubtedly well qualified to speak, and undoubtedly were selected because each had contributed significant research, the presence of such people may have foreclosed discussion of their work. The panel reports sometimes seemed to want only to preserve good feelings among the members by uncritically including everyone's contribution, with little concern for internal contradiction. The panel reports tended not to be carefully reasoned documents, but statements crafted to win support by minimizing overt conflict and criticism.

It was clear also to many panelists that "success" was measured by influencing the Commission to adopt the panel's recommendations. Because the game was to persuade, task panelists might have believed that being tentative in their recommendations would have resulted in undermining the force of a position. As we noted, a goodly number of the Commissioners were not professionals closely attuned to data based arguments. Forcefulness of presentation may have weighed more heavily than cautious "on the one hand . . ." arguments in that group.

If it is true that the Commission's methods of working (i.e., a highly politicized task environment, uncertain criteria, and a need to persuade) led to much less precise review and analysis, then the major loss for the future is that the three volumes of appendices are considerably less useful as technical resources for professionals, for political leaders and their staffs, and for the public than they might have been had the Commission's structure and its working formats been conceived in some different fashion.

When we do examine the more adequate reports, it seems that

each one was influenced by groups that already had established positions, and that had documentation of various kinds for those positions. The Task Panel on Women produced one of the better written, and more closely reasoned reports. It based its work on feminist assumptions, and as noted, its appendix included the entire list of resolutions passed at the 1977 National Women's Conference in Houston, a conference which made national news in part because representatives of traditionally oriented women's groups felt they had been left out. In recent years, feminists have been articulating positions in mental health. Female professionals have been creating a mental health literature based on feminist assumptions, and many have been active within the ranks of professional organizations pressing for change in the status of women within those organizations. When this opportunity arose, those with a feminist viewpoint had prepared materials to draw on, and in a situation in which speed was of the essence, those with prepared positions can carry the day because others have neither the time, nor the inclination to engage in extended critiques and analyses in the short working time.

Another Task Panel report of merit was the one produced by the group on Migrant and Seasonal Workers. This group was able to call on prepared documents and positions developed by advocacy groups and by numerous federal agencies. It acknowledged the assistance of the staff of the National Association of Farmworkers Organizations in producing their report.

The Task Panel on Legal and Ethical issues also had a forceful, well presented report. Influential members of the Task Panel had established well defined, well articulated positions long before the task panels ever met. NIMH, for example, had been supporting litigation and efforts to change state mental health laws, both within its own walls and through contracts with the American Bar Association, the Mental Health Law Project, and others (Kopolow et al., 1975). The group was an "establishment," composed of professionals, many of whom knew each other from other contacts, and who had previously articulated positions to draw on. We are not arguing that each group should begin *de novo*, but anyone with a prepared position can dominate a relatively brief conference under pressure to produce a report from busy members scattered around the country.

The character of the Task Panel reports is enlightening in another direction. In 1961, the Joint Commission felt that among the reasons mental health was underfunded and neglected was its lack of a broad-based political constituency. There was, in the years following the Second World War, a small but effective coalition of congressional leaders with interests in health and science, a politically savvy administrative elite within NIMH, with allies among the leadership of several professions, and an existing citizen's organization that lobbied effectively for mental health services (Foley, 1975).

It is a favorite strategem of administrative agency heads to spread the benefits of any funded program to as many different constituencies as possible, for then they become voices in support of a program when it comes up for congressional review (Wildavsky, 1964). Foley (1975) states that such a course of action was used knowingly and effectively by the NIMH leadership. In the course of developing NIMH research and training programs, and later the Community Mental Health Centers program, financial resources were distributed to all the states, to many different professional groups, to many different academic disciplines, and to many types of institutions. Foley, for example, believes that it is no accident that many of the CMHC's first appeared in the districts represented by legislators who served on congressional committees that made important decisions about mental health funding. In 1973 when mental health funds were threatened with impoundment by the Nixon administration, it was the National Council of Community Mental Health Centers, a group organized to deal collectively with the government about the status of funds and regulations governing them, which led the legal fight that forced Nixon to spend the funds Congress had appropriated (*National Council of Community Mental Health Centers* v *Weinberger*, 1973).

If the Joint Commission felt, in 1961, that there was no mental health constituency, it seems fair to say that there is now a broad constituency, but it is not composed of "grassroots" people, or even the consumers of services. The new political constituency is the set of providers of services and the research community that benefits economically from available funds. The very act of supporting training, research, and service has led to a demand for continued support from among the growing number of articulate and influential people who are the beneficiaries of programs. That constituency is evident in the care with which various Task Panels acknowledged that they had consulted and drawn upon the work of many existing groups, including committees of the American Psychiatric Association, the Children's Defense Fund, the National Association of State Mental Health Program Directors, the National Council of Community Mental Health Directors, the Mental Health Association, the American Nurses Association, the Mental Patients Liberation Front, and many, many similarly titled organizations. Not only would many of these groups have prepared positions on many topics, but they are potential supporters for governmental funding, if their interests are adequately represented. It was politically sensible to consult as many groups as possible, and to represent their positions if at all possible, even if to do nothing more than enhance the coalition in favor of funding in general. Under these circumstances, it is not surprising that critical appraisals were lacking.

We have not considered the ADAMHA bureaucracy as an organized interest group, but it too must be considered, for undoubtedly members of that group also have articulated positions which appeared in the President's Commission report as the judgments of the Commission. Foley (1975) noted that the community mental health policy was pursued for many years despite changes in political administrations. We must assume that today's bureaucrats are no less able in pursuing their policies than their predecessors.

Despite the deficiencies in the Task Panel reports, they nevertheless must be considered seriously because they reflect the viewpoints of organized, and less obviously organized, special interest groups and "establishments" which will press for their positions in whatever forum is available. We can expect that these positions will continue to influence legislation, policy, and administrative decisions concerning the distribution of funds. The future is in these documents not because of their basis in facts, but because they represent articulated positions of groups able to press in organized fashion for them.

The argument should not be misread. One can never expect such a thing as disinterested deliberation and decision making in the mental health world. I am not singling out the President's Commission. I believe the field should be sensitive to the issues I have raised here precisely because most work in public policy is not disinterested, data based, and neutral in its implications, although it might appear as such when presented in the guise of the deliberations of scientists and experts. What is surprising is not that such a politicized constituency exists, but how large and diverse it has now become.

The President's Commission Report. Just as we can tell something of the political constituencies for mental health services from the character of the Task Panel reports, so the Report to the President tells us something about the processes influencing mental health policies. While I shall point out some deficiencies in the Report, my criticisms are tempered by the knowledge that the art of policymaking is still crude, although it is not clear that experts on policy and planning would have produced any more valid set of recommendations. It may be that the collective judgment of wise, informed, intelligent people is the best we can expect. However, it is important to look at what was produced and how it was produced, or at least rationalized, for the Report went on to influence policy formation at the level of the Secretary of Health and Human Services (formerly HEW), and in many ways it is at the heart of the Carter administration's Mental Health Systems Act, passed by Congress.

The report itself is a brief document, totaling 57 pages of text and 21 pages of footnote and annotation. Interestingly, the footnotes and annotations do not document the source of the recommendations found in the body of the Report, but are elaborations of the recommendations. The Report has a brief introduction, with a generalized assertion of findings of fact, and then it makes its recommendations, each presumably deriving from the findings of fact. Each recommendation is preceded by a brief statement representing the analysis supporting the recommendation. The analysis can frequently be traced back to materials in a Task Panel Report, but often it consists of arguments or assertions about what would be desirable.

Before looking at its recommendations, we should look at what it didn't do, at least not in the Report itself. It did not review existing practices or state and federal legislation bearing on its areas of concern, although it may have assumed intimate familiarity with the Community Mental Health Centers Act and amendments. It did not deal in any detail with criticisms of existing practice, or of the role of government in relation to existing practice. It didn't evaluate alternatives in order to provide a detailed view of the advantages, disadvantages, costs and benefits, or values underlying the recommendations. Neither did it discuss issues of political and public acceptibility, problems in implementtation that might be anticipated, time perspectives, nor criteria for evaluation. It didn't consider any possible unintended consequences of its recommendations which in general were pragmatic and general, rather than specific. In a significant proportion of the recommendations, one could not be certain of what sort of program would fulfill the generalities expressed, what its cost would be, and what would be considered criteria of successful implementation in the short- as well as in the long-run. In many respects its mission might have been very limited both by the short period allotted it to report, and its view of itself as being constrained by what currently existed.

The Commission's basic thrust is that "mental health care of high quality and reasonable cost should be available to all who need it." It asserts that the overall demand for services may include nearly 15 percent of the population (p.8). To this end, the Commission asks a redress in the imbalance between physical and mental health expenditures, because so many are afflicted with mental health problems. While it is concerned about public and private financing of mental health services, its financing recommendations center on reforming the existing patchwork system, pending national health insurance legislation. (In confirmation of this view there is now a powerful, extended-provider constituency, the Commission supported insurance reimbursement for psychologists, social workers, and nurses with advanced degrees, and the inclusion of such qualified mental health practitioners for independent insurance reimbursement under national health insurance legislation. It also supported the freedom of choice concept in insurance legislation that has been so important in states requiring insurance reimbursement to nonmedical practitioners. Given the ongoing war between psychology and psychiatry in particular (see *Virginia Academy of Clinical Psychologists et al.* v *Blue Shield of Virginia* Civ. Action No. 78-0495-A. E.D. Va. April 9, 1979; reversed, 4th Cir. June 16, 1979; cert denied 49 LW 3617), the Commission's position represents significant support for nonmedical practitioners.) In the Commission's report, we have moved to the point where the supply of mental health services is conceived of as a right, and the financing of it as a public responsibility. Staying within the medical model, the Commission has asserted that a great many problems in living are the public's business.

Although the concepts of high quality and reasonable cost are central, they are unanalyzed in the Commission's report. No standards of quality are asserted, unless we look to its support of the Professional Standards Review Organization as a quality control device, and its mention of accrediting and licensing procedures. It does not endorse the latter moves toward professionalization, but it is clear that its thinking is influenced by professional standards of service delivery, and not by other humane considerations as such (see Levine, 1979). Perhaps the commission assumes that guaranteeing good professional quality will guarantee humane standards of care. It leaves this determination, however, in the hands of professional bodies, without any leavening influence of consumer participation or control. While in general we can believe that professional standards are motivated by humane considerations, I have also noted many ways in which professions have followed self-interest at the expense of their clients. The issues should not be foreclosed by failing to examine the underlying assumptions.

There is no analysis of the concept of reasonable cost. For example, issues of benefit-cost ratios and problems of estimating benefits for the aged, the very young, and the chronically disabled, as well as the costs and benefits of having a humane society, are not considered. The standard of cost comparison (when are costs unreasonable?) is not discussed, nor is there any consideration of the needs of the caretakers of the aged, the young, and the chronically disabled and dependent. The unanalyzed concept sounds good, but it conceals the tough questions. A commission consisting of high-minded and disinterested citizens might well have fostered a discussion of tough questions and might well have put the issues in front of the lay and professional public alike.

One of the most important aspects of the report, reflected in its recommendations for new service initiatives, is its emphasis on the concept of the unserved, underserved, and inappropriately served populations. It identifies these as children, adolescents, the elderly, racial and ethnic minorities, to a lesser extent women, and those with chronic mental illness. It also considers underserved geographic areas—rural communities and the inner cities. It proposes providing services for these groups directly by new funding initiatives for services, and indirectly, by providing training funds to increase the supply, of personnel trained to work in the priority areas, geographic and human. These recommendations are very much in keeping with policy statements reflected in NIMH documents over the last several years describing training, research, and service programs.

Although there are proposals for alleviating a problem, the problem is not closely analyzed. We do not know if services are available but populations don't use them for their own cultural reasons; whether the available services are not suitable to needs as members of the target populations perceive their own needs; whether the social costs of using services are too high; whether it is a matter of financial restraints, and if so, for which groups; whether it relates to the social and personal characteristics of providers vis à vis the recipients of service; or whether the types of training available in most existing training settings would be inappropriate for the underserved population. In an earlier chapter, we pointed out the mental health system has both an ameliorative and a social control function. The Commission has focused on the ameliorative function, as it should, but in neglecting the social control function, it may not allow for a thorough analysis that might have some chance of avoiding problems that emerge when ameliorative and social control functions are mixed, providing double-binding messages.

The failure to think through problems will result in recommendations and programs that are inherently self-defeating. For example, the recommendations for financing and quality of care emphasize professional standards of quality care. The bias toward reimbursement of professional services, with an emphasis on traditional professional standards, might well result in the provision of exactly those services, delivered in a manner and by types of personnel that led the President's Commission to feel concerned about under- and inappropriately served in the first place.

Recommendations for the care of the chronic patient similarly does not carefully consider the point made by the U.S. Senate Subcommittee on Long Term Care (1976) and the Comptroller General (1977) that the reimbursement formula for federal aid to the states was as much responsible for the unfortunate ways in which deinstitutionalization came about as any other single factor. Beyond the failure to see the contribution of federal welfare policies to the deinstitutionalization problem, there is little recognition of the problems of local government and private sector agencies in providing the community based services that were to have followed patients into the community. Moreover, the chronic population appears to be treated as an undifferentiated whole, with little understanding that differentiated services may be necessary. Fairweather et al. (1969) made the suggestion that we may need to consider legal statuses intermediate to fully independent and legally committed patients if we are to deal with the problems of the chronic client and at the same time satisfy the needs of communities. The Commission did not confront such issues.

Most important, the Commission did not really give any thought to the issues of a philosophy of care for chronic mental patients. What is the nature of the "good life" for the chronically disabled and dependent toward which we are aiming, and in what kind of settings may that vision of the good life best be fulfilled? What would be the cost of providing services that would fulfill the aims, and what is the political feasibility of paying for those services? And what of the caretakers of the chronically dependent? What constitutes the good life for them? How do we reward them and sustain them and prevent them from burning out or losing their humanity? The Commission seems to have adopted the thinking of the hastily mounted community support program, developed in response to congressional criticism that preceded the announcement of the community support program. The Commission missed the opportunity to take a fresh look at this enduring and vexing problem.

The Commission is rightly concerned about the fragmentation of our service system, if it can be called a system in any formal sense. Its plans call for coordination of state mental health plans with health plans developed through the Health Systems Agency planning process. The service system is composed of private sector agencies, local and state government supported agencies, and many of the support services—transportation, housing, income maintenance, vocational rehabilitation—come from outside the mental health and the health systems. The Commission's plan does not clearly come to terms with the fragmentation that violates the wholistic character of human need. Note also that while the Commission has as its goal the readjustment of imbalance between mental health and health expenditures, it is questionable that reliance on the medically dominated Health Systems Agency for planning will provide that balance.

The discussion of the needs for children and adolescent services does not consider the nature of those services. Are they for psychotherapeutic services, family therapy, or chemotherapy for children to reduce disruptive behavior in the schools? There is little or no discussion about the job market for adolescents in general and minority youth in particular, or about how secondary school programs relate or fail to relate to foreseeable needs. There is a new emphasis on competency testing in high schools. That emphasis may well reduce sharply the number of minority and poorer children achieving high school diplomas, or it may increase the number of older, disaffected children kept back because they failed to meet the school's standard of competency. What are the mental health and social implications of that trend in the schools? The Commission's clinical focus is entirely too narrow, and so misses the opportunity to be of much use.

Championing prevention probably reflects the most innovative of the Commission's recommendations. At this writing, it is not clear to what degree the recommendations will be followed, even though provisions for prevention programs are part of the Mental Health Systems Act. Albee (1979), one of the major proponents of prevention programs, has expressed concern that prevention will not fare well against the professional in-fighting he saw as the new legislation was being planned. However, just as the Joint Commission's Report in 1961 served as the rallying ground for the profound developments we have seen since its time, so the President's Commission report may also legitimate an area of concern, with the result that funds will be allocated and work supported. It may well be that when next the area of mental health is reviewed, the President's Commission Report may be seen as a benchmark for future progress, and the development of programs in prevention, if that comes to pass, may well be seen as a major consequence of the Commission's foresight.

Chapter 8

THE FUTURE OF
COMMUNITY MENTAL HEALTH
AND THE MENTAL HEALTH
SYSTEMS ACT (1980)

The future of community mental health will, in part, depend on the fate of the Mental Health Systems Act (PL 96–398), passed by Congress on October 7, 1980. It is difficult to predict the influence of the Act. Although it authorizes continuation of provisions to establish additional community mental health centers, and authorizes as much as $260 million in spending for new initiatives through fiscal 1984, a new administration has taken office, and a new Congress, highly conservative fiscally as predicted, has assumed office. Authorization for spending in legislation is one thing. Appropriation by the Congress for such spending is quite another. Funds cannot be spent until the Congress appropriates them by specific legislative action. In the past, mental health legislation had its friends in Congress, and in fact President Ford's veto of mental health appropriations in 1975 was actually overridden by the Democrat-controlled congress. Now the Senate is controlled by the Republican party, and it is unlikely that a Reagan veto would be seriously challenged. Nonetheless, it is still important to review the provisions of the new Act because it is very likely that some of them will be funded. And in any event, since its provisions reflect stable forces in the mental health sociopolitical context, undoubtedly there will be continuing efforts to see that all its provisions are funded and implemented in some degree. The remainder of this chapter is an examination of the pertinent provisions of the Mental Health Systems Act, showing their relationship to the President's Commission Report, and analyzing the significance of the provisions. (In view of the mood of the current Congress, we may be discussing ancient history.)

Community mental health centers. Section 101 of Title I of the Act contains a definition of a CMHC similar to the one under which previous centers were established, except that a newly established center need not provide the full range of services at once. Both new and currently funded CMHCs will be organized into mental health service areas (see below) rather than catchment areas. Each will provide: inpatient, emergency, and outpatient services; assistance to courts and other agencies; followup care for patients discharged from inpatient facilities; and consultation and education services to help develop new programs and coordinate existing ones, to publicize programs, and to assist in rape treatment, prevention, and control programs. Aftei the initial three years, each new center will also have to provide day care and partial hospitalization, a range of specialized services for children and the elderly, transitional and halfway-house services, and programs in prevention, treatment, and rehabilitation for alcoholism and drug abuse. Comprehensive services must be coordinated with those provided by other agencies in the mental health service area. Centers may provide the services themselves, or on contract with other agencies.

Services must be provided in a manner preserving human dignity, assuring the quality of care, and taking into account geographic, cultural, linguistic, and economic considerations. Each CMHC is required to have a governing body representative of the mental health service area, or if the program is operated by a governmental hospital, a representative advisory body. The Act further specifies a quality assurance program, integrated medical records, a staff professional advisory body to consult with the governing body, and when appropriate, a separate, identifiable administrative unit for consultation and education services.

Most of the requirements in the definition are familiar. They have been eased somewhat to make it easier for new centers to begin operations. Centers still receiving funding under the previous Act will continue to receive such funding. New centers will be organized under the provisions of the new Act. The Act authorizes a total of $105 million for fiscal 1982 through 1984 for new grants.

The state mental health authority and the mental health service areas. In order to coordinate mental health planning with medical health planning, catchment areas are now to be designated mental health service areas, and their boundaries are to conform or are to be contained within the boundaries of the medical health service areas established under the Public Health Service Act authorizing the Health Systems Agencies and areas for health planning. (Since the Health Systems Agencies may be discontinued by the Congress, this plan is also in jeopardy.) In order to facilitate the participation of state mental health authorities in community mental health work, the Act authorizes grants for administrative costs, planning, research, and evaluation, and for initiating patient's rights protection programs. The state departments of mental health may be allotted a total of $45 million over the three fiscal years ending September 30, 1984.

Provisions for funding of administrative units within state departments of mental health were made in recognition that in the past, federal programs have tended to bypass the state departments, and in recognition that coordinated services require the participation of state mental health authorities. The funds were also authorized in recognition that states have become the chief sponsors for "graduating" centers (i.e., those that have completed their periods of eligibility for federal funding), and are now heavily involved in community mental health programs that the states were previously seen as opposing.

The state mental health authority is given additional power in the Act. All grant applications for funds under most of the titles in the Act must be passed through the state mental health authority. It passes along its judgment of the rank order of priority for funding for each grant when it transmits it to the Secretary. The Secretary of HHS can also enter into exclusive contracts with a state authority (§305) to develop, monitor, and implement a deinstitutionalization plan, to develop case management services, regulations for community residences, for community education, and for in-service education to improve the skills of those working with the chronically mentally ill in the community.

In order to be eligible to receive funds (see Title III), the state mental health authority must develop a state mental health services plan in consultation with the statewide Health Coordinating Council, which prepares statewide health plans under the Public Health Service Act. The statewide plan must be consistent with the mental health provisions of the state health plan, which by virtue of §303, amending the Public Health Service Act, must have mental health provisions.

While the government thus gives considerable power to the state mental health authority, it also specifies what the federal government wants to cover in a plan (§302). The state mental health plan must contain provisions for meeting the needs of institutional employees displaced by deinstitutionalization; mental health service areas congruent with health service areas must be established; and a needs assessment and evidence of how the plan will meet the needs of the underserved priority populations are necessary. Each state plan must deal with geographic, cultural, linguistic, and economic barriers to the delivery of mental health services. Each state plan must also identify existing legal rights of mental patients in that state, and indicate what steps it will take to remove deficiencies in that state's laws. Each state is asked to give assurances that the entire state will be covered adequately, and that the state will make provision to continue services provided by local agencies when their eligibility for federal support ends.

In addition to the statewide plan, the Act has additional provisions for monitoring and enforcement. Section 315 calls for performance contracting, although the legislative history (p.60) makes it clear that the Congress does not expect to overburden mental health facilities with demands for documentation. If there has been a "substantial and persistent failure" (§321) to implement the state's mental health program, or on the part of any agency to implement provisions of a grant or contract for mental health services, the Secretary may, after suitable hearings, discontinue payments. In other words, although the new Act gives a considerably greater role to state mental health authorities, and continues roles for local service providers, its provisions indicate that the federal government may exercise a great deal of control to see that the basic purposes and terms of the Act, and grants and contracts under it, will be fulfilled. It is not clear how tightly the standard "substantial and persistent failure" will be applied in reviewing programs, and it may be that performance review, except in the most blatant cases, will prove relatively ineffectual in dealing with more and even less subtle conversions of federal funds to business as usual.

New service plans. Following the President's Commission recommendation, new funds are authorized to support grants for services to the chronically mentally ill (§202), children and adolescents (§203), and the elderly and other priority populations (§204). The bulk of the newly authorized funds are designed for programs for the chronically mentally ill, but substantial amounts are also allocated to the other services. Existing CMHCs will have priority in applying for programs to meet the new service objectives. However, provision is made for other agencies to sponsor specialized programs as well. Programs for children and adolescents must be coordinated with services provided by the schools and other agencies in relation to PL 94–142, the so-called mainstreaming legislation, and other federally authorized service programs for this population. There are similar requirements for coordination of programs provided to the elderly and other priority populations.

Designed to provide new service initiatives following the recommendations of the President's Commission, these efforts are also designed to bring about more productive interaction among programs, agencies, and services which have so far functioned separately. Whether the mandate will be effective remains to be seen. At any rate, the new directives provide a basis for agencies generally divorced from each other to begin talking seriously about cooperation.

Cooperation between mental health and health care centers. Section 206 provides for grants to link mental health services to ambulatory care centers, nursing homes, health facilities, and programs and intermediate care facilities. The Act employs the granting mechanism to provide care to the large number of the elderly who now reside in nursing homes and related facilities. It may also facilitate mental health service agreements between existing general health care facilities and CMHCs, furthering the aim of coordinating care.

Prevention. Section 208 makes provision for grants for projects for the prevention of mental illness and for the promotion of positive mental health. The projects do not have to be routed through the state mental health authority, although they should be consistent with efforts aimed at prevention in other health care legislation. A total of $21 million was authorized for the three fiscal years ending September 30, 1984. Section 325 of Part E of Title III requires that the director of NIMH designate an administrative unit within NIMH responsible for overseeing programs in prevention. While the most ardent proponents of prevention were far from winning a full victory, and while they were very far from the target goal of gaining 10 percent of mental health funds dedicated to prevention, the proverbial camel's nose is under the NIMH tent. The possibilities for future efforts are now there, however weak the fledgling program appears.

In 1979, The Surgeon General of the United States sponsored a conference to establish objectives in prevention in national health care. The topics included: hypertension, family planning, pregnancy and infant health, immunization, sexually transmitted diseases, toxic agent control, occupational safety and health, accident prevention and injury control, flouridation, surveillance and control of infectious diseases, smoking and health, alcohol and drug abuse, nutrition, physical fitness and exercise, and stress. In each of these areas, the technical problems were less the necessity to develop biologically oriented information, and more the necessity to develop behavioral, educational, sociological, and politically feasible approaches. Even if prevention in mental health is a long way from achieving full partnership in the panoply of mental health services, preventive thinking is currently pervasive in the health fields, and is built into the operation of the new, and as yet slowly developing health maintenance organizations (HMOs). (See *Professional Psychology,* 1979, *10,* No. 4, entire issue.)

The presence of provisions for programs in prevention should give one pause about the time scale for program development, and for the persistence of ideas through the vicissitudes of time, political administrations, and fads and fancies in the field. Prevention was championed by some members of the Joint Commission some twenty to twenty-five years earlier, and some of their views have now influenced the formal statement of public policy as embodied in federal legislation. Whether one is encouraged or discouraged by the pace of change will depend upon one's temperament, and ability to maintain an olympian historical perspective in viewing developments in the mental health field.

Minority affairs. Title IV, §401, establishes an office for an Associate Director for Minority Concerns within NIMH. The Associate Director, now evidently a line item in the NIMH budget, is directed to oversee minority concerns in research, training, service, and support programs. It is not an affirmative action office. Rather it is to be concerned with promoting the substantive concerns of minority groups within all NIMH programs.

Mental health rights and advocacy. Title V welcomes a newcomer to the formally funded mental health family. The Title includes a mental patients Bill of Rights and urges each state to review and revise its mental health laws in light of the statement. The legislation adopts many of the recommendations of the President's Commission and its Task Panel on Legal and Ethical Issues. In part, the legislative language reflects the court victories since 1966. Given our federal system, the Congress can only urge state legislatures to bring their laws into compliance, but it can encourage such compliance with funding incentives.

Given the prominent place in the legislation of the patient's Bill of Rights, imaginative attorneys will undoubtedly find ways of using its terms in pressing litigation, especially with facilities receiving federal funds. Given that state mental health authorities are likely to be defendants in such cases, it may be that state legislators will be receptive to changes to modernize their laws.

The Act (§502) provides grants for services to protect and to advocate for the rights of mentally ill individuals. These grants are limited to agencies independent of those providing treatment or services to the mentally ill. Having forestalled a conflict of interest, the legislation ensures political control over the watchdog. The governor of each state designates the entity to receive funds if it is an agency of government, or recommends the agency if a public or nonprofit corporation. If applications are made by agencies other than those designated by the governor, or recommended by him, the Secretary of HHS is obligated to notify the governor of the application and give the governor and other interested parties the opportunity to comment on the application at a hearing. Whether such advocacy organizations will actively operate as patients' rights watchdogs will depend on the degree to which the governor of a state controls the facility to limit the embarrassment it might cause an incumbent. Using one's machiavellian imagination, one could foresee one interest group funding an activist advocacy agency in a backward state to promote active litigation and so harrass the party in power.

Funds in the amount of $10 million were authorized for the first year with the amount rising to $15 million by the third year. While the amount is relatively small, if as little as half went to create new full-time positions, some 200 lawyers would become active in the field, and since they would be bringing legal action against many state agencies and local service providers, those agencies will also be in need of legal counsel versed in mental health law. The nucleus for a small industry is present here, and we should follow the developments with interest.

Rape services. Interest in the serious problem of rape, largely promoted by activist women's groups, is given recognition under §101(b)(v) in the requirement that consultation and education services relate to rape prevention, treatment, and control programs. More importantly, under Title VI, modest funds are allocated for continued research efforts into a variety of aspects of the problem of rape. The Secretary of HHS will be assisted in allocating funds for the studies by an advisory council, a majority of whom must be women, and who will be reimbursed for their consulting services. A still larger amount of money is allocated to public and private groups providing services to rape victims. This Title contains the major recognition of women's mental health needs, in keeping with the low profile given women's needs in the President's Commission Report.

Indian tribes. Indian tribes receive consideration in §308. Tribes or intertribal organizations, in recognition of their unique legal status, may apply directly to the Secretary, bypassing state mental health authorities. However, applications must be submitted to the Indian Health Service for transmittal, and for certification that the application is consistent with the Tribal Specific Health Plan. While Indians are thus accorded some special status in the legislation, no funds are specifically set aside for Indian problems.

Innovative projects. The legislation (§207) allots some funds to the Secretary of HHS to support innovative projects in training, retraining, or redeployment of personnel adversely affected by changes in the mental health service delivery system. The funds may also be used to support any other innovative project with national significance in the delivery of mental health services or in the use of mental health personnel. In any fiscal year, the Secretary can use 5 percent of appropriated monies available for purposes of most of the sections of the Act. If all authorized funds were appropriated, the Secretary could spend about $8 million on such projects. These grants may be made directly by the Secretary, in any amount, upon direct application to the Secretary, and without the approval of the state mental health authority. While the legislation attaches some strings to the expenditure of the funds, the Secretary is given a small amount of relatively free funds to support projects of interest to the Secretary, in agencies of interest to the Secretary.

ITERATION AND REITERATION

The new legislation seems to have something for everyone. It gives state mental health authorities more power and a little more money. It centralizes control of planning for service delivery in the health system, not an unmitigated blessing from some viewpoints. The legislation endorses the community mental health concept, and encourages states to make plans to fund "graduating" centers. The requirements make it easier to start new CMHCs, a recommendation of the President's Commission. To meet criticisims of the cruel aspects of deinstitutionalization, the legislation authorizes the expenditure of a good deal more money on services in the community for the chronically mentally ill. In addition, it provides funds for new services targeted to the previously underserved priority populations. The interests of a variety of constituencies—minorities, Indians, women, advocates of prevention, community mental health center workers, displaced employees within institutions—are recognized in one way or another.

Most of the Act's provisions can be traced back to the recommendations of the President's Commission on Mental Health. However, their proposals were not new. Many of them reflected policies that were discernible in pronouncements and requirements coming from NIMH and ADAMHA. Programs for the underserved, for example, were given priority for funding long before the President's Commission reported. It is my opinion that the persistent attention to the problem of the underserved reflected democratic and humanistic values of members of the federal bureaucracy, who because of their staying power and their ability to control information, pressed for priority to the underserved. I do not believe there is much organized political pressure to provide for the underserved. There are good, data based arguments for paying attention to the needs of those populations. In this instance, I think that those we sometimes denigrate by the term bureaucrat have served the forces of conscience. I note the role of the federal bureaucracy because they too are actors in the drama, and certain of their interests also affect the shape of mental health programs.

Most of the time, mental health policies are shaped by provider constituencies, and those provider constituencies have important socioeconomic stakes in continued funding. The battle for insurance reimbursement is currently preempting professional attention. However, the battle for expanded services in the public sector is equally important. The social problems of those in the priority populations, and those we characterize as the chronically mentally ill, will not magically disappear. And organized groups of those who earn their livings from the delivery of services will, understandably, act to protect their jobs. The President's Commission Task Panel Reports should continue to be consulted, despite many unfortunate inadequacies, because they contain the subtle blend of data, argument, and enlightened self-interest that will power future political effort.

It is too early to predict the fate of the new legislation. This chapter was written just after the 1980 presidential election, and just after the Reagan administration took office. The administration acted, in the words of Senator Daniel P. Moynihan, to wipe out thirty years of social legislation with the stroke of a pen. The final budget has not yet been passed by the Congress. At this writing it appears as if mental health programming will be turned back to the states by means of block grants with few federal strings attached. However, I do not think the provisions of the Act will be totally abandoned by either the federal government or by the states. There was support in Congress for mental health legislation. The Congress expressed its satisfaction with the progress that had been made in the legislative history accompanying the committee reports on the House and Senate bills. That expression of satisfaction can be attributed, in part, to the successful present-ation of the case for CMHCs by the ADAMHA bureaucracy to the Congress. In the past, the CMHC program fared reasonably well, despite all the talk of budget cuts and despite hostile admin-istrations. About 400 centers were established during the Nixon and Ford years, and over 200 more during the Carter administra-tion. Moreover funds go to all 52 states, as well as to the District of Columbia, Puerto Rico, Guam, and the Virgin Islands.

Mental health legislation still has friends in Congress. Senator Edward Kennedy, although no longer in a majority post in the Senate, is still an influential figure, favorably disposed not only on ideological grounds, but perhaps also because the CMHC concept is a major legacy to the nation from his brother. The policy of moving away from the state hospital and toward community based services had its origins in the 1950s, almost from the very inception of NIMH. One can see considerable continuity of policy since the Joint Commission's report in 1961.

Now, of course, the movement has developed a substantial constituency among mental health service providers, and these groups are more articulate and more organized than twenty years ago. As of February 1978, there were 70,496 employees of feder-ally funded CMHCs, and an unknown additional number providing contract services to meet the requirement of a comprehensive service delivery program (U.S. Senate Committee on Labor and Human Resources, 1980). Spending by the states on mental health services far outweighs the amount spent by the federal government, and the Act's provisions encourage states to take new initiatives in services. Mental health programs are tightly woven into the system, and will be with us for a long time to come, despite the prospects for a short-range funding drought.

The Act takes seriously some of the problems of fragmentation, and has recognized these, if it has not adequately confronted them. Whether the approach that mandates cooperation and provides some incentives for cooperation will be sufficient to overcome structural fragmentation remains to be seen. Based on the experience of recent years, we can expect that the waters will be churned, and in some places some workable models may emerge.

However, there are forces pulling toward the status quo, and even a return to a reliance on the institution and the medical model. The pressures of community resistance to community placement, and the continued dependence on third-party payments, may well pull services back to heavy utilization of inpatient facilities. The Act contains within it the strengths and weaknesses of governmental action. It reveals a partial willingness to come to grips with emergent problems without jettisoning what has promise and value. However, it also reveals the need, so characteristic of the political system, to give a little something to everyone. Although there is recognition of the system problem, it is not clear that palliative measures will come to grips with the system problem definitively.

Having said that our expectations should be limited by the complexity of the political system, I may not have said very much that was not obvious to everyone except mental health professionals busily engaged in doing their best to serve their clients, and experiencing political problems as irrational noises in the system. It is not noise in the system. Political issues are integral in the context within which mental health services are devised and delivered. The issues have been with us, as this book has tried to show, since the first mental hospitals were established in their modern form in mid-nineteenth century. Political issues set the stage for the development of federal involvement in mental health from the First World War on, and they influenced the federal involvement after the Second World War. As the last few chapters have shown, political issues, like the poor, will always be with us. The error is to deny the problem or try to ignore it.

The field of mental health by no means belongs exclusively to the professional mental health workers no matter how fervently we wish it. The reality is that public mental health services are necessarily influenced by their social, political, and economic context. We are no different than persons and associations concerned with agriculture, commerce, defense, energy, and other major segments of socioeconomic reality. The political system is there. Our view of ourselves as disinterested scientist-professionals distorts the reality of our existence. It may be that the lesson of the President's Commission and its effect on subsequent legislation is its clarification of our tasks for the future. It may be that it is our task as professionals, and as teachers of the next generation of professionals, to engage in consciousness raising so that political science, law, and economics become as much parts of the mental health curriculum, for many if not for all, as abnormal psychology or psychotherapy.

We should not give up the scientist-professional model, nor should we depart from our service ideal, but the needs of the future, both of the profession and of its clients, will depend upon a much more sophisticated and self-conscious appreciation of the contexts within which we live and work than has characterized our fields in the past.

References

Abramson, M.F. The criminalization of mentally disordered behavior: Possible side effects of a new mental health law. *Hospital and Community Psychiatry*, 1972, *23*, 101-5.

Addington v State of Texas 99 S.Ct. 1804 (1979).

Albee, G.W. *Mental health manpower trends.* New York: Basic Books, 1959.

Albee, G.W. Preventing prevention. *APA Monitor*, 1979, *10*, No. 5 (May), p. 2.

Albers, D.A., & Pasewark, R.A. Involuntary hospitalization. Surrender at the courthouse. *American Journal of Community Psychology*, 1974, *2*, 287-89.

Albers, D.A., Pasewark, R.A., & Smith, T.C. Involuntary hospitalization: The social construction of danger. *American Journal of Community Psychology*, 1976, *4*, 129-32.

Altmeyer, A.J. *The formative years of Social Security.* Madison: University of Wisconsin Press, 1966.

Anthony, W.A. *The principles of psychiatric rehabilitation.* Amherst, Mass.: Human Resource Development Press, 1979.

Anthony, W.A., Buell, G.J., Sharratt, S., & Althoff, M.E. Efficacy of psychiatric rehabilitation. *Psychological Bulletin*, 1972, 78, 447-56.

Arnhoff, F.N. Social consequences of policy toward mental illness. *Science*, 1975, *188*, 1277-81.

Aviram, U., & Segal, S. From hospital to community care: The change in the mental health treatment system in California. *Community Mental Health Journal*, 1977, *13*, 158-67.

Bachrach, D.L. (NIMH) Deinstitutionalization: An analytical review and sociological perspective. Washington, D.C.: DHEW Publication No. (ADM) 76-351, 1976.

Baker, F. Planning and the environment of a community mental health center. *Psychiatric Quarterly*, 1972, *46*, 95–108.

Baker, F. The living human service organization: Applications of general systems theory and research. In H.W. Demone and D. Harshbarger (Eds.) *A handbook of human service organizations*. New York: Behavioral Publications, 1974.

Baker, F., & Broskowski, A. The search for integrality: New organizational forms for human service systems. In D. Harshbarger and R. Maley (Eds.) *Behavior analysis and system analysis: An integrative approach to mental health programs*. Kalamazoo, Mich.: Behaviordelia, 1974.

Baker, F., Broskowski, A., & Brandwein, R. System dilemmas of a Community Health and Welfare Council. *Social Service Review*, 1973, *47*, 63–80.

Bartley v *Kremens* 402 F. Supp. 1039 (E.D. Pa. 1975).

Bass, R.D. *Sources of funds, Federally funded Community Mental Health Centers, 1971*. Washington, D.C.: DHEW, NIMH, OPPE, Biometry Branch, Survey and Reports Section. Statistical Note 91, 1973.

Baxtrom v *Herold* 383 U.S. 107 (1966).

Becker, H.S. *Outsiders: Studies in the sociology of deviance*. New York: Free Press of Glencoe, 1963.

Beers, C.W. *A mind that found itself*. New York: Longmans, Green, 1908.

Bell, N.W., & Spiegel, J.P. Social psychiatry: Vagaries of a term. *Archives of General Psychiatry*, 1966 *14*, 337–45.

Berman, N., & Hoppe, E.W. Halfway house residents: Where do they go? *Journal of Community Psychology*, 1976, *4*, 259–60.

Birnbaum, M. Right to treatment. *American Bar Association Journal*, 1960, *46*, 499.

Blatt, B. *Exodus from pandomonium*. Boston, Mass.: Allyn and Bacon, 1970.

Blatt, B., & Kaplan, F. *Christmas in purgatory: A photographic essay on mental retardation*. Boston, Mass.: Allyn & Bacon, 1966.

Bleuler, E. *Dementia praecox or the group of schizophrenias*. New York: International Universities Press, 1950.

Bloom, B.I. *Community mental health. A general introduction*. Monterey, Cal.: Brooks-Cole, 1977.

Board of Managers of the State Lunatic Asylum. 30th Annual Report of the Managers of the State Lunatic Asylum. Utica, New York, for the year 1872. Albany, N.Y.: Argus, 1873.

Bockoven, J.S. *Moral treatment in community mental health*. New York: Springer, 1972.

Bradley, V., & Clarke, G. (Eds.). *Paper victories and hard realities: The implementation of the legal and constitutional rights of the mentally disabled*. Washington, D.C.: The Health Policy Center, Georgetown University, 1976.

Braginsky, B.M., Braginsky, D.D., & Ring, K. *Methods of madness. The mental hospital as a last resort.* New York: Holt, Rhinehart and Winston, 1969.

Brand, J.L. The National Mental Health Act of 1946: A retrospect. *Bulletin of the History of Medicine,* 1965, *39*, 231–45.

Broderick, A. Justice in the books or justice in action: An involuntary approach to involuntary hospitalization for mental illness. *Catholic University Law Review,* 1971, *20*, 547–701.

Brooks, A.D. *Law, psychiatry and the mental health system.* Boston: Little, Brown, 1974.

Brownmiller, S. *Against our will. Men, women and rape.* New York: Simon & Schuster, 1975.

Butler, R.N. *Why survive? Being old in America.* New York: Harper & Row, 1975.

Byers, E.S., Cohen, S., & Harshbarger, D.D. Impact of aftercare services on recidivism of mental health patients. *Community Mental Health Journal,* 1978, *14*, 26–34.

Califano v *Goldfarb* 430 U.S. 199 (1977).

Caplan, R.B. *Psychiatry and the community in nineteenth century America.* New York: Basic Books, 1969.

Carpenter, J.O., & Bourestom, N.C. Performance of psychiatric hospital discharges in strict and tolerant environments. *Community Mental Health Journal,* 1976, *12*, 45–51.

Christenfeld, R., & Haveliwala, Y.A. Patients' views of placement facilities: A participant observer study. *American Journal of Psychiatry,* 1978, *135*, 329–32.

Chu, F.D., & Trotter, S. *The madness establishment: Ralph Nader's study group report on the National Institute of Mental Health.* New York: Grossman, 1974.

Clarke, S.H. & Koch, G.G. Juvenile court: Therapy or crime control and do lawyers make a difference? *Law and Society Review,* 1980, *14*, 263–308.

Cohen, C.I., Sichel, W.R., & Berger, D. The use of a mid-Manhattan hotel as a support system. *Community Mental Health Journal,* 1977, *13*, 76–83.

Cohen, F. The function of the attorney and the commitment of the mentally ill. *Texas Law Review,* 1966, *44*, 424–67.

Cole, J.O. & Gerard, R.W. *Psychopharmacology. Problems in evaluation.* Washington, D.C., National Academy of Sciences. National Research Council, 1959.

Coll, B.D. *Perspectives in public welfare* (U.S. Department of Health, Education & Welfare, SRS, Office of Research, Demonstrations and Training. Intramural Research Division). Washington, D.C.: U.S. Government Printing Office, 1969.

Colten, S.I. Community residential treatment strategies. *Community Mental Health Review*, 1978, *3(1)*, 16–21.

Cometa, M.S., Morrison, J.K., & Ziskoven, M. Halfway to where? A critique of research on psychiatric halfway houses. *Journal of Community Psychology*, 1979, *7*, 23–27.

Committee on Interstate and Foreign Commerce. *Mental Health Systems Act*. Report No. 96–977, House of Representatives, 96th Congress, 2nd Session. Washington, D.C.: U.S. Government Printing Office, 1980.

Comptroller General of the United States. Report to the Congress. Returning the mentally disabled to the community: Government needs to do more. Washington, D.C.: Comptroller General of the U.S., January 7, 1977.

Connery, R.H., Backstrom, C.H., Deener, D.R., Friedman, J.R., Kroll, M., Marden, R.H., McCleskey, C., Meekison, P., & Morgan, J.A., Jr. *The politics of mental health*. New York: Columbia University Press, 1968.

Covington v Harris 419 F. 2d 617 (D.C. Cir. 1969).

Crown, S. "On Being Sane in Insane Places": A comment from England. *Journal of Abnormal Psychology*, 1975, *84*, 453–55.

Dain, N. *Concepts of insanity in the United States, 1789–1865*. New Brunswick, N.J.: Rutgers University Press, 1964.

Davis, A.E., Dinitiz, S., & Pasamanick, B. The prevention of hospitalization in schizophrenia. Five years after an experimental program. *American Journal of Orthopsychiatry*, 1972, *42*, 375–88.

Davis v Watkins 384 F. Supp. 1196 (N.D. Ohio 1974).

Dawkins, M.P., & Dawkins, M.P. A program for the treatment of post-hospitalized mental patients in a low-income Black community. *Journal of Community Psychology*, 1978, *6*, 257–62.

Decker, G., & Shealy, A.E. Rates of admission to state mental hospitals in Alabama for counties with mental health clinics versus those without clinics. *Journal of Community Psychology*, 1973, *2*, 54–56.

Delaney, J.A., Seidman, E., & Willis, G. Crisis intervention and the prevention of institutionalization: An interrupted time series analysis. *American Journal of Community Psychology*, 1978, *6*, 33–46.

Denner, B. Returning madness to an accepting community. *Community Mental Health Journal*, 1974, *10*, 163–72.

Deutsch, A. *Shame of the states*. New York: Harcourt Brace, 1948.

Deutsch, A. *The mentally ill in America*. 2nd ed. New York: Columbia University Press, 1949.

Dewey, R. The jury law for commitment of the insane in Illinois (1867–1893) and Mrs. E.P.W. Packard its author, also later developments in lunacy legislation in Illinois. *American Journal of Insanity*, 1913, *69*, 571–84.

Dixon v *Attorney General of The Commonwealth of Pennsylvania* 325 F. Supp. 966 (M.D. Pa. 1971).

Dixon v *Weinberger* 405 F. Supp. 974 (D.D.C. 1975).

Doidge, J.R., & Rodgers, C.W. Is NIMH's dream coming true? Wyoming centers reduce state hospital admissions. *Community Mental Health Journal,* 1976, *12,* 399–404.

Donaldson, K. *Insanity inside out.* New York: Crown, 1976.

Ellis, N.R. The Partlow case: A reply to Dr. Roos. *Law and Psychology Review,* 1979, *5*(Fall) 15–49.

Emde, R.N. From state hospital to community psychiatry: Problems in two kinds of communities. *Community Mental Health Journal,* 1967, *3,* 203–10.

England, J.M. Dr. Bush writes a report: "Science—The Endless Frontier." *Science,* 1976, *191,* 41–47.

Ennis, B.J. *Prisoners of psychiatry. Mental patients, psychiatrists and the law.* New York: Harcourt Brace Jovanovich, 1972.

Ennis, B.J., & Siegel, L. *The rights of mental patients.* New York: Avon Books, 1973.

Ennis, B.J., & Dubose, E.I., Heineman, B.W., Jr., & Friedman, R.R. Brief for the respondent. In the Supreme Court of the United States, October term, 1974, 74–8, J.B. O'Connor, petitioner, Kenneth Donaldson, respondent. Washington, D.C.: Mental Health Law Project, 1975.

Ennis, B.J., & Litwack, T.R. Psychiatry and the presumption of expertise: Flipping coins in the courtroom. *California Law Review,* 1974, *62,* 693–752.

Fairweather, G.W., Sanders, D.H., Cressler, D.F., Maynard, H., & Bleck, D.S. *Community life for the mentally ill.* Chicago, Ill.: Aldine, 1969.

Felix, R.H. *Mental illness—Progress and prospects.* New York: Columbia University Press, 1967.

Fleming, G.M. Historical survey of the educational benefits provided veterans of World War II by the Servicemen's Readjustment Act of 1944. Unpublished Ed.D. Thesis, University of Houston, 1957.

Foley, H.A. *Community mental health legislation.* Lexington, Mass.: D.C. Heath, 1975.

Foucault, M. *Madness and civilization.* New York: Pantheon, 1965.

Fuchs, V.R. *The service economy.* New York: National Bureau of Economic Research, Columbia University Press, 1968.

Galbraith, J.K. *The affluent society.* Boston: Houghton, 1958.

In re Gault 387 U.S. 1 (1967).

Gideon v *Wainwright* 372 U.S. 335 (1963).

Gish, L. *Reform at Osawatomie State Hospital.* Lawrence: University Press of Kansas, 1972.

Goffman, E. *Asylums.* New York: Doubleday, 1961.

Goldhamer, H., & Marshall, A.W. *Psychosis and civilization: Two studies in the frequency of mental disease.* Glencoe, Ill.: The Free Press, 1953.

Goldman, H. Conflict, competition, and coexistence: The mental hospital as parallel health and welfare systems. *American Journal of Orthopsychiatry,* 1977, *47,* 60–65.

Goldstein, A.S. *The insanity defense.* New Haven, Conn.: Yale University Press, 1967.

Goplerud, E. Unexpected consequence of deinstitutionalization of the mentally disabled elderly. *American Journal of Community Psychology,* 1979, *7,* 315–28.

Goshen, C.E. *Documentary history of psychiatry.* New York: Philosophical Library, 1967.

Gottesfeld, H. Alternatives to psychiatric hospitalization. *Community Mental Health Review,* 1976, *1,* 1–10.

Gove, W.R. Societal reaction as an explanation of mental illness. *American Sociological Review,* 1970, *35,* 873–84.

Graziano, A.M. Clinical innovation and the mental health power structure: A social case history. *American Psychologist,* 1969, *23,* 10–18.

Grob, G.N. *The state and the mentally ill.* Chapel Hill: University of North Carolina Press, 1966.

Grob, G.N. *Mental institutions in America.* New York: The Free Press, 1973.

Gupta, R.K. New York's Mental Health Information Service: An experiment in due process. *Rutgers Law Review,* 1971, *25,* 405–35.

Gusfield, J.R. *Symbolic crusade: Status politics in the American Temperance Movement.* Urbana: University of Illinois Press, 1963.

Gustafson, T. The controversy over peer review. *Science,* 1975, *190,* 1060–66.

Halderman v *Pennhurst State School and Hospital* 451 F. Supp. 233 (E.D. Pa. 1978) Aff'd. Civ. No. 78-1999 (3d Cir. 1979); rev'd and remanded 49 LW 4363 (1981).

Henry, J. *Culture against man.* New York: Random House, 1963.

HEW Task Force. Report of the HEW Task Force on Implementation of the Report to the President from the President's Commission on Mental Health. Washington, D.C.: DHEW Publication No. (ADM) 79-848, 1979.

Hiday, V.A. Reformed commitment procedures: An empirical study in the courtroom. *Law and Society Review,* 1977, *11,* 651–66.

Horwitz, M.J. *The transformation of American law 1780–1860.* Cambridge, Mass.: Harvard University Press, 1977.

Hostica, C. Summary process. Unpublished paper. SUNY Buffalo School of Law and Jurisprudence, 1974.

Hoyt, W.B. & Hopkins, D. Saturation of certain areas of Erie County with social service-oriented, community based halfway houses. Report prepared by Office of New York State Assemblyman, William B. Hoyt, 1976.

Jackson v *Indiana* 406 U.S. 715 (1972).

Jahoda, M. *Current concepts of positive mental health.* New York: Basic Books, 1958.

Johnson, P.E. *A shopkeeper's millennium. Society and revivals in Rochester, New York*, 1815–1837. New York: Hill & Wang, 1978.

Joint Commission on Mental Health of Children. *Crisis in child mental health: Challenge for the 1970's.* New York: Harper & Row, 1969.

Joint Commission on Mental Illness and Health. *Action for mental health.* New York: Basic Books, 1961.

Kanner, L. *A history of the care and study of the mentally retarded.* Springfield, Ill.: Charles C Thomas, 1964.

Kaplan, H.M., & Bohr, E.H. Change in the mental health field? *Community Mental Health Journal*, 1976, *12*, 244–51.

Kennedy, J.F. Mental illness and mental retardation. Message from the President of the United States relative to mental illness and mental retardation. House of Representatives, 88th Congress, 1st Session, Document No. 58, February 5, 1963.

Kesey, K. *One flew over the cuckoo's nest.* New York: Viking Press, 1962.

Kirby, M.W., Polak, P.R., & Deever, S. On treating the insane in sane places. *Journal of Community Psychology*, 1977, *5*, 380–87.

Kirk, S.A., & Therrien, M.E. Community mental health myths and the fate of former hospitalized patients. *Psychiatry*, 1975, *38*, 209–17.

Kittrie, N.N. *The right to be different. Deviance and enforced therapy.* Baltimore, Md.: The Johns Hopkins Press, 1971.

Koenig, P. The problem that can't be tranquilized. *The New York Times Magazine*, May 21, 1978, *58*, 14–17.

Kopolow, L.E., Brands, A.B., Barton, J.L., & Ochberg, F.M. Litigation and mental health services. DHEW Publication No. (ADM) 76–261. Washington, D.C.: NIMH, 1975.

Kropotkin, P. *Mutual aid: A factor of evolution.* New York: New York University Press, 1972. (Originally published 1899).

LaFave, H.F., Stewart, A., & Grunberg, F. Community care of the mentally ill: Implementation of the Saskatchewan plan. *Community Mental Health Journal*, 1968, *4*, 37–46.

Lake v *Cameron* 364 F. 2d 657 (D.C. Cir. 1966).

Lamb, H.R. Rehabilitation in community mental health. *Community Mental Health Review*, 1977, *2*, 3–8.

Lamb, H.R., & Edelson, M.B. The carrot and the stick: Inducing local programs to serve long term patients. *Community Mental Health Journal*, 1976, *12*, 137–44.

Lamb, H.R. & Goertzel, V. Discharged mental patients—Are they really in the community? *Archives of General Psychiatry*, 1971, *24*, 29–34.

Landsberg, G. & Hammer, R. Possible programmatic consequences of community mental health center funding arrangements: Illustrations based on inpatient utilization data. *Community Mental Health Journal*, 1977, *13*, 63–67.

Lehmann, S., Mitchell, S., & Cohen, B. Environmental adaptation of the mental patient. *American Journal of Community Psychology*, 1978, *6*, 115–24.

Lemert, E. *Social pathology: A systematic approach to the theory of sociopathic behavior*. New York: McGraw-Hill. 1951.

Lessard v Schmidt 349 F. Supp. 1078 (E.D. Wis. 1972). 94 S.Ct. 713, 1974.

Levine, A. & Schweber-Koren, C. Jury selection in Erie County. Changing a sexist system. *Law and Society Review*, 1976, *11*(1), 43–55.

Levine, M. Some postulates of community psychology practice. In F. Kaplan and S.B. Sarason (Eds.), *The Psycho-Educational Clinic Papers and Research Studies*. Springfield, Mass.: Massachusetts Department of Mental Health, 1969.

Levine, M. Some postulates of practice in community psychology and their implications for training. I. Iscoe and C.D. Spielberger (Eds.), *Community psychology, perspectives in training and research*. New York: Appleton-Century-Crofts, 1970.

Levine, M. Congress (and evaluators) ought to pay more attention to history. *American Journal of Community Psychology*, 1979, *7*, 1–16.

Levine, M. *From state hospital to psychiatric center. The implementation of planned organizational change*. Lexington, Mass.: D.C. Heath, 1980.

Levine, M. & Bunker, B.B. (Eds.). *Mutual Criticism*. Syracuse, N.Y.: Syracuse University Press, 1975.

Levine, M., & Levine, A. *A social history of helping services*. New York: Appleton-Century-Crofts, 1970.

Levine, M., & Perkins, D.V. Social setting interventions and primary prevention: Comments on the Report of the Task Panel on Prevention to the President's Commission on Mental Health. *American Journal of Community Psychology*, 1980, *8*, 147–58.

Levitt, L.I., Brownlee, W.H., & Lewars, M.H. A model project in community mental health: Consultation to an urban welfare center serving a single-room occupancy hotel. *Community Mental Health Journal*, 1968, *4*, 494–98.

Longmate, N. *The workhouse*. New York: Random House, 1974.

Lottman, M.S. Paper victories and hard realities. In V. Bradley and G. Clarke (Eds.), *Paper victories and hard realities: The implementatation of the legal and constitutional rights of the mentally disabled.* Washington, D.C.: The Health Policy Center, Georgetown University, 1976.

Luckey, J.W., & Berman, J.T. Effects of a new commitment law on involuntary admissions and service utilization patterns. *Law and Human Behavior,* 1979, *3*(3), 149–62.

Marx, A.J., Test, M.A., & Stein, L.I. Extrahospital management of severe mental illness. *Archives of General Psychiatry,* 1973, *29,* 505–11.

McClain, R.E., Silverstein, A.B., Hubbell, M., & Brownlee, L. Comparison of the residential environment of a state hospital for retarded clients with those of various types of community facilities. *Journal of Community Psychology,* 1977, *5,* 282–89.

McGarry, A.L., Curran, W.J., Lipsitt, P.D., Lelos, D., Schwitzgebel, R., & Rosenberg, A.H. Competency to stand trial and mental illness. DHEW Publication No. (ADM) 74–103. Washington, D.C.: NIMH Center for Studies of Crime and Delinquency, 1973.

McNees, M.P., Hannah, J.T., Schnelle, J.F., & Bratton, K.M. The effects of aftercare programs on institutional recidivism. *Journal of Community Psychology,* 1977, *5,* 128–33.

Meehl, P.E., & Rosen, A. Antecedent probability and the efficiency of psychometric signs, patterns or cutting scores. *Psychological Bulletin,* 1955, *52,* 194–216.

Menninger, W.C. Lessons from military psychiatry for civilian psychiatry. *Mental Hygiene,* 1946, *30,* 577–82.

Meyer, N.G. Legal status of inpatient admissions to state and county mental hospitals, United States, 1972. Statistical Note 105, Division of Biometry, Survey and Reports Branch, NIMH, 1974.

Michaux, M.H., Prium, R.J., Dasinger, E.M., & Prium, B.A. Day hospital admissions: A unique treatment group. *Journal of Community Psychology,* 1973, *1,* 427–30.

Miller, K.S. *Managing madness.* New York: Macmillan, 1976.

Millon, T. Reflections on Rosenhan's "On being sane in insane places." *Journal of Abnormal Psychology,* 1975, *84,* 456–61.

Monahan, J. The prevention of violence. In J. Monahan (Ed.) *Community mental health and the criminal justice system.* New York: Pergamon Press, 1976.

Monahan, J. Strategies for an empirical analysis of prediction of violence in emergency civil commitment. *Law and Human Behavior,* 1977, *1*(4), 363–72.

Monahan, J., & Wexler, D.B. A definite maybe: Proof and probability in civil commitment. *Law and Human Behavior,* 1978, *2*(1), 37–42.

Morse, S.J. Crazy behavior, morals, and science: An analysis of mental health law. *Southern California Law Review*, 1978, *51*(4), 527–54.
Moscowitz, I. The effectiveness of day hospital treatment: A review. *Journal of Community Psychology*, 1980, *8*, 155–64.
Moss, F.E., & Halamandaris, V.J. *Too old, too sick, too bad.* Germantown, Md.: Aspen Systems Corporation, 1977.
Murphy, J. Psychiatric labelling in cross-cultural perspective. *Science*, 1976, *191*, 1019–28.
Musto, D.F. *The American disease. Origins of narcotic control.* New Haven, Conn: Yale University Press, 1973.

Nathan, V.M. The use of masters in institutional reform litigation. *Toledo Law Review*, 1979, *10* (winter), 419–64.
National Council of Community Mental Health Centers v *Weinberger,* 361 F. Supp. 897 (D.D.C. 1973).
National Institute of Mental Health. Community living arrangements for the mentally ill and disabled. Issues and options for public policy. Proceedings of a Working Conference, NIMH, Ramada Inn, Rosslyn, Virginia, September 22–24, 1976. Washington, D.C.: HEW, USPHS, ADMHA, 1976.
New York State Commission in Lunacy. *1st Annual report of the State Commission in Lunacy for the year 1889.* Albany, N.Y.: Wynkoop, Hollenbeck, Crawford, 1896.
Nevid, J.S., Capurso, R., & Morrison, J.K. Patients' adjustment to family-care as related to their perceptions of real-ideal differences in treatment environments. *American Journal of Community Psychology*, 1980, *8*, 117–20.
NYARC v *Rockefeller* 357 F. Supp. 752 (E.D. NY 1973).
Note. Implementation problems in institutional reform litigation. *Harvard Law Review*, 1977, *91*, 428–63.
Note Case. The *Wyatt* case. Implementation of a judicial decree ordering institutional change. *Yale Law Journal*, 1975, *84*, 1338–79.

O'Connor v *Donaldson* 422 U.S. 563 (1975).
O'Gorman, M. *Every other bed.* Cleveland: World Publishing Co., 1956.
Ordronaux, J. *Commentaries on the lunacy laws of New York and on the judicial aspects of insanity at common law and in equity including procedure as expounded in England and the United States.* Albany, N.Y.: J.D. Parsons, 1878.

Packard, E.P.W. *Modern persecution of insane asylums unveiled as demonstrated by the Investigation Committee of the legislature of Illinois.* Vol. I. *Modern persecution of married women's liabilities* as demonstrated by the action of the Illinois legislature. Vol. II. Hartford, Conn.: Case, Lockwood, & Brainard, 1875. (New York: Arno Press, New York Times, 1973, facsimile edition).

Parham v J.L. and J.R. 99 S.Ct. 2493 (1979).

Parry, H.J., Balter, M.B., Mellinger, G.D., Cisin, I.H., & Manheimer, D.L. National patterns of psychotherapeutic drug use. *Archives of General Psychiatry*, 1973, *28*, 769–83.

Parry-Jones, W.L. *The trade in lunacy.* London: Routledge & Kegan Paul, 1972.

Pasamanick, B., Scarpitti, F.R., & Dinitz, S. *Schizophrenia in the community: Experimental studies in the prevention of hospitalization.* New York: Appleton-Century-Crofts, 1967.

Perlman, N. The worker's perspective. In V. Bradley and G. Clarke (Eds.), *Paper victories and hard realities. The implementation of the legal and constitutional rights of the mentally disabled.* Washington, D.C.: Health Policy Center, Georgetown University, 1976.

Perry, J. Community placement of chronic psychiatric patients. Unpublished qualifying paper, Ph.D. Program in Clinical-Community Psychology, SUNY at Buffalo, 1978.

Pierce, F. Veto message. Congressional Globe, 33rd Congress, 1st Session, May 3, 1854, 1061–63.

Pinel, P. *A treatise on insanity.* (Translated by D.D. Davis.) Sheffield, England: Cadell and Davies, 1806.

Platt, A.M. *The child savers. The invention of delinquency.* Chicago, Ill.: University of Chicago Press, 1969.

Polak, P., & Jones, M. The psychiatric non-hospital: A model for change. *Community Mental Health Journal*, 1973, *9*, 123–32.

Polansky, N. Medical vs sociological models of change. Review of M. Levine and A. Levine, A social history of helping services. *Contemporary Psychology*, 1971, *16*, 211–12.

Polier, J.W. *A view from the bench: The Juvenile Court.* New York: National Council on Crime and Delinquency, 1964.

Pound, R. Law in books and law in action. *American Law Review*, 1910, *44*, 12–36.

Poythress, N.G. Psychiatric expertise in civil commitment: Training attorneys to cope with expert testimony. *Law & Human Behavior*, 1978, *2*(1), 1–24.

President's Commission on Mental Health. *Report to the President.* Vol. I. Washington, D.C.: U.S. Government Printing Office, Stock Number 040-000-00390-8, 1978a.

President's Commission on Mental Health. *Task Panel Reports.* Vols. II, III, IV. Appendix. Washington, D.C.: U.S. Government Printing Office, Stock Numbers 040-000-00391-6; 040-000-00392-4; 040-000-00393-2; 1978b.

Purvis, S.A., & Miskimins, R.W. Effects of community follow-up on post-hospital adjustment of psychiatric patients. *Community Mental Health Journal*, 1970, *5*, 374–82.

Radinsky, T.L. Transfer completion rates and treatment modality. *Journal Community Psychology*, 1976, *4*, 239–45.

Ray, I. *A treatise on the medical jurisprudence of insanity.* (1838). Cambridge, Mass.: Harvard University Press, 1962.

Redick, R.W. Patterns in use of nursing homes by the aged mentally ill. Washington, D.C.: DHEW, PHS, ADMHA, NIMH, Division of Biometry, Survey and Reports Branch, Statistical Note 107, June, 1974.

Reisman, J.M. *A history of clinical psychology.* New York: Irvington Publishers, 1976.

Reissman, C.K., Rabkin, J.G., & Struening, E.L. Brief versus standard psychiatric hospitalization: A critical review of the literature. *Community Mental Health Review*, 1977, *2*(1), 3–10.

Riordan, W.L. *Plunkitt of Tammany Hall.* New York: McClure, Phillips, 1905.

Robbins, E., & Robbins, L. Charge to the community: Some early effects of a state hospital system's change of policy. *American Journal of Psychiatry*, 1974, *131*, 641–45.

Rog, D.J., & Raush, H.L. The psychiatric halfway house: How is it measuring up? *Community Mental Health Journal*, 1975, *11*, 155–62.

Roos, P. Custodial care for the "subtrainable"—Revisiting an old myth. *Law and Psychology Review*, 1979, *5*(Fall), 1–14.

Roosens, E. *Mental patients in town life. Geel—Europe's first therapeutic community.* Beverly Hills, Cal.: Sage Publications, 1979.

Rosen, G. *Madness in society.* Chicago: University of Chicago Press, 1968.

Rosenhan, D.L. On being sane in insane places. *Science*, 1973, *179*, 250–58.

Rosenhan, D.L. The contextual nature of psychiatric diagnoses. *Journal of Abnormal Psychology*, 1975, *84*, 462–74.

Rothman, D.J. *The discovery of the asylum.* Boston: Little, Brown, 1971.

Rouse v Cameron 373 F. 2d 451 (D.C. Cir. 1966).

Sarason, S.B. *The psychological sense of community. Prospects for a community psychology.* San Francisco: Jossey-Bass, 1974.

Sarason, S.B. Community psychology and the anarchist insight. *American Journal of Community Psychology*, 1976, *4*, 246–61.

Sarason, S.B. The nature of problem solving in social action. *American Psychologist*, 1978, *33*(4), 370–80.

Sarason, S.B. *Psychology misdirected.* New York: The Free Press, 1981.

Sarason, S.B., & Doris, J. *Psychological problems in mental deficiency.* 4th Ed. New York: Harper & Row, 1969.

Sarason, S.B., Levine, M., Goldenberg, I.I., Cherlin, D.L., & Bennett, E.M. *Psychology in community settings.* New York: Wiley, 1966.

Sauber, S.R. State planning of mental health services. *American Journal of Community Psychology*, 1976, *4*, 35–45.

Scheff, T.J. *Being mentally ill.* Chicago, Ill.: Aldine, 1966.

Scheff, T.J. (Ed.). *Labeling madness.* Englewood Cliffs, N.J.: Prentice-Hall, 1975.

Schulberg, H.C., & Baker, F. The caregiving system in community mental health programs: An application of open-systems theory. *Community Mental Health Journal,* 1970, *6,* 437–46.

Schulberg, H.C., & Baker, F. *The mental hospital and human services.* New York: Behavioral Publications, 1975.

Schulberg, H.C., Becker, A., & McGrath, M. Planning the phasedown of mental hospitals. *Community Mental Health Journal,* 1976, *12,* 3–12.

Selye, H. General adaptation syndrome and diseases of adaptation. *Journal Clinical Endocrinology,* 1946, *6,* 117–28.

Sinclair, A. *Era of excess. A social history of the prohibition movement.* New York: Harper & Row, 1964.

Sindberg, R.M. A fifteen year follow-up study of community guidance clinic clients. *Community Mental Health Journal,* 1970, *6,* 319–24.

Souder v *Brennan* 367 F. Supp. 808 (D.D.C. 1973).

Southard, E.E., & Jarrett, M.C. *The kingdom of evils.* New York: Macmillan, 1922.

Specht v *Patterson* 386 U.S. 605 (1967).

Spitzer, R.L. On pseudoscience in science, logic in remission, and psychiatric diagnoses: A critique of Rosenhan's "On being sane in insane places." *Journal of Abnormal Psychology,* 1975, *84,* 442–51.

Stein, A. *Adult homes: The nursing home scandal of the 1980's.* New York State Assembly, Albany, New York, February 23, 1976.

Stevens, R., & Stevens, R. *Welfare medicine in America.* New York: The Free Press, 1974.

Stone, A.A. *Mental health and law: A system in transition.* DHEW Publication No. (ADM) 75-176. Washington, D.C.: National Institute of Mental Health, Center for Studies in Crime and Delinquency, 1975.

Stone, A.A. Recent mental health litigation: A critical perspective. *American Journal of Psychiatry,* 1977, *134,* 273–79.

Stouffer, S.A., Lumsdaine, A.A., Lumsdaine, N.H., Williams, R.M., Jr., Smith, M.B., Janis, I.L., Star, S.A., & Cottrell, L.S., Jr. *The American soldier: Combat and its aftermath.* Princeton, N.J.: Princeton University Press, 1949.

Stouffer, S.A., Suchman, E.A., DeVinney, L.C., Star, S.A., & Williams, R.M., Jr. *The American soldier. Adjustment during Army life.* Princeton, N.J.: Princeton University Press, 1949.

Surgeon General's Ad Hoc Committee on Planning for Mental Health Facilities. Planning of facilities for mental health services. Washington, D.C.: U.S. DHEW Public Health Service Publication No. 808, January 1961.

Szasz, T.S. The uses of naming and the origin of the myth of mental illness. *American Psychologist,* 1961, *16,* 59–65.

Szasz, T.S. *The myth of mental illness.* New York: Harper & Row, 1961.

Szasz, T.S. *Law, liberty and psychiatry.* New York: Macmillan, 1963.

Szasz, T.S. *The manufacture of madness.* New York: Harper & Row, 1970.

Task Panel on Costs and Financing. Report of the Task Panel on Cost and Financing. Submitted to The President's Commission on Mental Health. In Task Panel Reports Submitted to the President's Commission on Mental Health, Appendix Vol. II. Washington, D.C.: U.S. Government Printing Office, Stock No. 040-000-00392-6, 1978.

Task Panel on Legal and Ethical Issues Report. In Task Panel Reports Submitted to the President's Commission on Mental Health. Vol. IV. Appendix. Washington, D.C.: U.S. Government Printing Office, Stock No. 040-000-00393-2, 1978.

Task Panel on Rural Mental Health. Report of the Task Panel on Rural Mental Health submitted to the President's Commission on Mental Health. In Task Panel Reports Submitted to the President's Commission on Mental Health, Appendix Vol. III. Washington, D.C.: U.S. Government Printing Office, Stock Number 040-000-00393-4, 1978.

Test, M.A., & Stein, L.I. Practical guidelines for the community treatment of markedly impaired patients. *Community Mental Health Journal,* 1976, *12,* 72–82.

Tucker, G. The progress of the United States in population and wealth. In E.C. Rozwenc (Ed.), *Ideology and power in the age of Jackson.* Garden City, N.Y.: Anchor Books, 1964. (Originally published 1855.)

Tuckman, J., & Lavell, M. Patients discharged with or against medical advice. *Journal Clinical Psychology,* 1962, *13,* 177–80.

Turner, J.E., Stone, G.B., & TenHoor, W. *The community support program: A draft proposal.* Washington, D.C.: Mental Health Services Support Branch, Division of Mental Health Service Programs, NIMH, January 10, 1977.

U.S. Bureau of the Census Statistical Abstract of the United States: 1976 (97th Edition). Washington, D.C., 1976.

U.S. Senate Committee on Labor and Human Resources. *Mental Health Systems Act.* Report No. 96–712, 96th Congress, 2nd Session, Washington, D.C.: U.S. Government Printing Office, 1980.

U.S. Senate Subcommittee on Long Term Care of the Special Committee on Aging. *The role of nursing homes in caring for discharged mental patients (and the birth of a for-profit boarding home industry).* Supporting paper No. 7, Washington, D.C.: U.S. Government Printing Office, 1976.

Vannicelli, M., Washburn, S.L. & Scheff, B.J. Partial hospitalization—
Better but why and for whom? *Journal Community Psychology,*
1978, *6,* 357–65.
Veroff, J., Feld, S., & Gurin, G. *Americans view their mental health.*
New York: Basic Books, 1960.
Virginia Academy of Clinical Psychologists et al. v *Blue Shield of
Virginia.* Civ. No. 78–0495–A (E.D. Va.) April 9, 1979; reversed
4th Cir. June 16, 1979; cert. denied 49 LW 3617.
Vladeck, B. *Unloving care.* New York: Basic Books, 1980.

Wald, P.M., & Friedman, P.R. Brief of American Orthopsychiatric
Association, American Psychological Association, Federation of
Parents Organizations for the N.Y. State Mental Institutions, Na-
tional Association for Mental Health, National Association for
Retarded Citizens, National Association of Social Workers and
National Center for Law and the Handicapped as *Amici Curiae* in
support of Appellees. In the Supreme Court of the United States,
No. 75–1064, Jack B. Kremens et al., Appellants v Kevin Bartley et
al. Apellees. Washington, D.C.: Mental Health Law Project, 1976.
Warner, A.G. *American charities.* (Revised by M.R. Collidge) 3rd Ed.
New York: Thomas T. Crowell, 1919.
Warren, C.B. Involuntary commitment for mental disorder: The applica-
tion of California's Lanterman-Petris-Short Act. *Law and Society
Review,* 1977, *11,* 629–50.
Weiner, B. "On being sane in insane places": A process (attributional)
analysis and critique. *Journal of Abnormal Psychology,* 1975, *84,*
433–41.
Weiner, D.B. The apprenticeship of Philippe Pinel: A new document,
"Observations of Citizen Pussin on the insane." *American Journal
of Psychiatry,* 1979, *136,* 1128–34.
Weinman, B., Sanders, R., Kleiner, R., & Wilson, S. Community based
treatment of the chronic psychotic. *Community Mental Health
Journal,* 1970, *6,* 13–21.
Welsch v *Likins* 373 F. Supp. 487 (D. Minn. 1974).
Wenger, D.L. & Fletcher, C.R. The effect of legal counsel on admissions
to a state mental hospital: A confrontation of professions. *Journal
of Health and Social Behavior,* 1969, *10,* 66–72.
Wildavsky, A. *The politics of the budgetary process.* Boston: Little,
Brown, 1964.
Willer, B. Scheerenberger, R.C., & Intagliata, J. Deinstitutionalization
and mentally retarded persons. *Community Mental Health Re-
view,* 1978, *3*(1), 3–12.
Windle, C., Bass, R.D., & Taube, C.A. PR aside: Initial results from
NIMH's Service Program Evaluation Studies. *American Journal
Community Psychology,* 1974, *2,* 311–27.
In re Winship, 397 U.S. 358 (1970).

Winters, E.E. Adolph Meyer and Clifford Beers 1907–1910. *Bulletin of the History of Medicine*, 1969, *43*, 414–43.

Witkin, M.J. Provisional patient movement and selective administrative data, state and county mental hospitals, inpatient services by state: United States, 1976 Mental Health Statistical Note No. *153*. NIMH, Division of Biometry and Epidemiology, Survey and Reports Branch, August 1979.

Witte, E.E. *The development of the Social Security Act*. Madison: University of Wisconsin Press, 1962.

Witten, M., Kerr, M., & Turque, C. State abandons mentally ill to city streets. *Village Voice*, October 31, 1977, *22*, 1, 2, 29.

Wolkon, G.H., Karmen, M., & Tanaka, H.T. Evaluation of a social rehabilitation program for recently released psychiatric patients. *Community Mental Health Journal*, 1971, *7*, 312–22.

Woodward, B., & Armstrong, S. *The brethren: Inside the Supreme Court*. New York: Avon, 1979.

Wyatt v *Aderholt*. See *Wyatt* v *Stickney* (1972).

Wyatt v *Ireland II*, Civ. No. 3195-N (M.D. Ala. 1979).

Wyatt v *Stickney*, 325 F. Supp. 781, 784 (M.D. Ala. 1971).

Wyatt v *Stickney*, 344 F. Supp. 373, 387 (M.D. Ala. 1972), aff'd *sub nom. Wyatt* v *Aderholt* 303 F. 2d 1305 (5th Cir. 1974).

Ziskin, J. Coping with psychiatric and psychological testimony. In A.D. Brooks (Ed.), *Law, psychiatry and the mental health system*. Boston: Little, Brown, 1974.

Zitrin, A., Hardestry, A.S., Burdock, E.I., & Drossman, A.J. Crime and violence among mental patients. *American Journal Psychiatry*, 1976, *133*, 142–49.

Zusman, J. Some explanations of the changing appearance of psychotic patients. *International Journal Psychiatry*, 1967, *3*, 216–37.

Name Index

Subject Index